Joyce and
Kent Fry

HANDBOOK OF MARITAL THERAPY

A Positive Approach to Helping Troubled Relationships

APPLIED CLINICAL PSYCHOLOGY

Series Editors: Alan S. Bellack and Michel Hersen
University of Pittsburgh, Pittsburgh, Pennsylvania

PARTIAL HOSPITALIZATION: A Current Perspective
Edited by Raymond F. Luber

HANDBOOK OF MARITAL THERAPY: A Positive Approach to Helping Troubled Relationships
Robert P. Liberman, Eugenie G. Wheeler, Louis A.J.M. deVisser, Julie Kuehnel, and Timothy Kuehnel

---

A Continuation Order Plan is available for this series. A continuation order will bring delivery of each new volume immediately upon publication. Volumes are billed only upon actual shipment. For further information please contact the publisher.

HANDBOOK OF MARITAL THERAPY

A Positive Approach to Helping Troubled Relationships

Robert P. Liberman
University of California
Los Angeles, California
and
Camarillo State Hospital
Camarillo, California

Eugenie G. Wheeler
Oxnard Community Mental Health Center
Oxnard, California

Louis A. J. M. de Visser
Loyola-Marymount University
Los Angeles, California
and
Santa Clara High School
Oxnard, California

Julie Kuehnel
University of California
Los Angeles, California
and
California Lutheran College
Thousand Oaks, California

and

Timothy Kuehnel
Camarillo State Hospital
Camarillo, California
and
University of California
Los Angeles, California

PLENUM PRESS • NEW YORK AND LONDON

Library of Congress Cataloging in Publication Data

Main entry under title:

Handbook of marital therapy.

Bibliography: p.
Includes index.
1. Marriage counseling. 2. Family therapy. I. Liberman, Robert Paul
HQ10.M372 362.8'2 79-9103
ISBN 0-306-40235-1

A Division of Plenum Publishing Corporation
227 West 17th Street, New York, N.Y. 10011

Printed in the United States of America

Foreword

In the treatment of marital problems, behaviorally oriented and communication oriented approaches have been in conflict and seen as contrasting and unlikely bed partners. Many therapists, focusing on communication skills, have felt that behaviorists were too structured and uncaring; on the other hand, behaviorists have considered humanistic therapists as being "touchy-feely," vague, and unfocused. However, in the *Handbook of Marital Therapy*, Liberman, Wheeler, de Visser, and the Kuehnels have wedded these two potent approaches into an integrated framework that makes them loving bed partners.

With over a decade of experience in applying behaviorally oriented treatment to couples, Liberman and his co-authors have developed an educational model that focuses on teaching specific communication skills to couples. The communication skills they describe have been used extensively in all types of marital therapy, regardless of the therapist's theoretical orientation.

The unique contribution of this book is that the authors provide a step-by-step approach to teaching these communication skills within a behavioral framework. Each chapter guides the therapist through the many issues and problems confronting him or her as a change agent. This highly readable book is enhanced by a liberal use of case examples. Emphasis is given to homework and structured sessions that focus on increasing specific communication skills in a sequential manner. The advantages of working with couples in a group setting are discussed, and concrete suggestions on how to manage these groups are clearly presented.

Liberman and his co-authors are to be commended for their effective blending of communication skills and behavioral therapy. This book provides a clear and concise descriptive guide for therapists and marriage counselors on how to enrich marital relationships. Most mental health professionals working with couples could benefit from this integrated approach to marital therapy.

David H. Olson

University of Minnesota
St. Paul, Minnesota

Preface

The methods described in this handbook derive from the field of behavior therapy and social learning theory. The authors have adapted the basic principles of behavior and human learning into techniques useful for helping married couples change. This work began in 1966, when the first author began treating married couples and families at the Massachusetts Mental Health Center in Boston. His work accelerated in 1971, when he became associated with the Oxnard Community Mental Health Center and joined with the second author in offering marital therapy to the numerous couples in conflict who sought assistance at the mental health center. The format and methods changed and were refined as the authors gained experience. Much of the refinement was carried out during 1972–1975, when the first author was granted funds for the Behavioral Analysis and Modification Project in Community Mental Health, an applied research project supported by the Mental Health Services Research and Development Branch of the National Institute of Mental Health (Grant No. MH 19880). Many of the details and tips in carrying out the methods described in this handbook derive from our experience in training 1,000 mental health professionals in 60 community mental health centers across the United States as part of a dissemination grant from the National Institute of Mental Health (Grant No. MH 26207).

A few innovators in behavioral marital therapy were particularly influential with the authors. We have borrowed heavily, in terms of conceptual understanding of marital conflict and satisfaction, assessment, and treatment, from Richard B. Stuart, A. Jack Turner, Robert Weiss, Gerald Patterson, Hyman Hops, Gary Birchler, Nathan Azrin, Barry Naster, and R. Jones. Our use of "core symbols" and contingency contracting derives from Stuart's work. The exercise entitled "Catch Your Spouse Doing or Saying Something Nice" was developed by Turner.

The fantasy fulfillment and reciprocity awareness exercises were described by Azrin, Naster, and Jones. Our emphasis on "love days," recreation, and marital activities was primed by the work of Weiss, Patterson, Hops, and Birchler. The fruits of these pioneers' work are clearly seen in the methods described in our handbook, and we owe them a very large professional and intellectual debt of gratitude.

The authors also wish to express their appreciation to Annelisa Romero, editor for the Department of Psychiatry and Behavioral Sciences, Neuropsychiatric Institute, UCLA, for her exceptionally skillful editorial scrutiny and suggestions.

ROBERT P. LIBERMAN
EUGENIE G. WHEELER
LOUIS A. J. M. DE VISSER
JULIE KUEHNEL
TIMOTHY KUEHNEL

Contents

Introduction

This treatment manual is a "how-to-do-it" guide for those in the helping professions who are actively concerned with the needs and problems of married or soon-to-be married couples. The treatment methods described in this manual cannot and should not be applied by individuals who have had little or no clinical experience. This is not a "cookbook" to be followed in a mechanical way. Experienced therapists who possess basic therapeutic attributes, such as warmth, empathy, interview skills, sensitivity, and positive regard for their clients, can put the approach described in this book to effective use. The detailed methods will be learned and applied more rapidly by professionals who are comfortable with an active, structured, and operational style of working with clients. However, all therapists and counselors—whatever their clinical style or theoretical orientation—will be able to adapt the techniques in this manual to their own work with couples.

People who can make use of this book include:

1. Marriage and family counselors who are interested in adding new and effective techniques to their clinical repertoires
2. Practicing mental health clinicians, such as psychiatrists, psychologists, social workers, and nurses, who must decide whether individual and/or marital therapy is appropriate for a particular client and then must offer the preferred alternative or make an appropriate referral
3. Pastoral counselors and other clergy who are called upon to assist couples with marital problems or who offer marital enrichment courses to their congregations or communities as part of their ministry
4. Probation officers, high school counselors, and other social service personnel who often must understand and cope with family and marital problems in the course of helping their clients and students
5. College and high school instructors or counselors who teach courses in marriage and family living

MARITAL THERAPY: WHAT AND FOR WHOM?

The therapy and training methods described in this manual can be used with couples experiencing moderate or severe marital conflict and stress, such as those who are on the verge of separation and divorce. Couples having problems communicating with each other and those resorting to punishing modes of interaction can benefit from the type of marital therapy illustrated in this book. This manual can also be used for couples with relatively minor marital problems who are looking for "growth" opportunities to make an "OK" relationship better. Such couples are often bored, feeling stifled, or taking each other for granted.

The methods for acquiring the communication, problem-solving, and family activity skills needed for marital improvement and satisfaction are highly structured and goal-oriented. These procedures may be utilized in individual, conjoint, or group therapy formats. The exercises and activities in this guide to marital therapy are based on our experiences as therapists in schools and universities, social agencies, mental health centers, and private practice. Research and evaluation studies conducted by the authors and by others have validated the effectiveness of these procedures. At the end of this book is an annotated bibliography of research publications that may be perused for more detailed documentation of the efficacy of our procedures. We did not want to dilute the clinical utility of the application portion of this manual with references or descriptions of supporting research; hence, these are reserved to the annotated bibliography. We do feel that enough convincing objective research has been done to warrant the widespread clinical adoption of the techniques reported in this book. Indeed, we would not have written this book or recommended the procedures had not sufficient scientific evidence accumulated to support their use. Social learning principles provided the foundation for these procedures, but a pragmatic concern for using "whatever works" guided their development and integration. In developing a workable marital therapy, we were not overly concerned with the relative partial contributions to treatment outcome made by each of the components of the treatment "package" nor with the theoretical purity of the "package."

Jay Haley (1963) has said that "marital therapy has not developed because of theory; it appears that people were struggling to find a theory to fit practice" (p. 214). Consequently, a number of "schools" of marital and family therapy exist that have different assumptions, languages, emphases, treatment techniques, treatment structures, and views of psychopathology or needs for growth. Setting the ideologies aside, we are struck by the common intervention focus of these various forms of marital therapy. All stress the importance of clear communication; accurate, empathic listening; the constructive expression of feelings; and the need for conflict resolution and problem-solving strategies for couples experiencing difficulty in their relationships. The social learning or behavioral approach to marital therapy described in this manual addresses each of these needs and thus shares a great deal with other forms of marital therapy, even though it stems from a different tradition. Consequently, several of the components of the procedures explained in this manual are not unique to the behavioral paradigm but are shared with avowedly "nonbehavioral" forms of marital therapy.

The general goals of our approach to marital therapy are to increase the couples' recognition, initiation, and acknowledgment of pleasing interactions; to decrease the couples' aversive interactions; to train the couple to communicate effectively; and to teach the couples to use contingency contracting for negotiating the resolution of persistent problems and dissatisfactions. The procedures described in this manual follow a behavioral counseling model, which emphasizes:

- Precise goal setting
- Measuring and monitoring progress
- Practicing desired behaviors
- Shaping small steps in adaptive directions
- Reinforcing progress
- Generalizing gains made in the clinic or office by the couples to their home environment

ORGANIZATION OF THE MANUAL

Chapter 1, "General Guidelines and Principles," provides an overview of the general process and techniques of behavioral marriage counseling. It also discusses the principles and basic assumptions behind these techniques and briefly covers the empirical evidence on which they are based.

Chapter 2, "Getting Started," describes the planning activities that must be carried out prior to commencing marital therapy. Topics covered include: recruiting clients and obtaining referrals, involving the reluctant partner, screening and selecting appropriate clients, increasing clients' motivation, setting positive therapeutic expectations, and contracting for services. These topics are covered for both conjoint and group forms of marriage therapy.

Chapter 3, "Planning Recreational and Leisure Time," focuses on patterns of recreational and leisure-time activities that are typically present in good marriages. A conceptual framework assists the therapist in guiding couples to more closely approximate satisfying patterns of recreational and leisure-time activities.

Chapter 4, "Communicating: Awareness of Reciprocity," focuses on the importance of couples' becoming more aware of the pleasing and caring exchanges in their relationship. A series of exercises is presented that can increase the partners' skills in asking for, giving, and receiving behaviors and events that can please each other. Homework assignments are provided that can increase the occurrence of these pleasing behavioral exchanges on a day-to-day basis.

Chapter 5, "Communicating: The Arts of Listening and Effectively Expressing Feelings," provides the therapist with a framework for teaching couples to express feelings directly and spontaneously. A most important component in this chapter is helping partners learn how to express negative and angry feelings in a nonaggressive or noncoercive manner.

Chapter 6, "Giving and Getting: Marital Contracts," covers the use of contingency contracting as a method of problem solving and resolving differences through negotiation and compromise. Chapters 3 through 6 are similar in that each chapter takes up the rationale and techniques for facilitating particular forms of marital interaction or communication skills. In addition, a series of step-by-step exercises and examples is provided to assist the therapist in teaching couples new patterns of interactions.

Chapter 7, "Ending," describes the termination process. Topics covered include how to structure the final sessions, arranging follow-up and booster sessions, referring for additional help, and recycling.

Chapter 8, "Solving Special Problems," provides suggestions for dealing with problems that occasionally occur in this form of therapy. Suggestions are given for handling couples who are reluctant to engage in role-play exercises, reacting to partners who do not complete their homework assignments, and dealing with resistance to a structured approach.

Chapter 9 is a summary of the manual, and Chapter 10 provides some suggested therapy session outlines for individual couples and for couples' groups. The last section is an annotated bibliography for professionals and clients.

Throughout these chapters, numerous examples are provided to illustrate marital therapy with couples experiencing a variety of problems. In addition, a case example based on a composite of couples we have worked with is used as a connecting thread throughout the manual. This example is referred to in each of the chapters to further illustrate the process of acquiring interaction skills and problem solving that typical couples go through as they proceed from awareness to awkward utilization, to more natural use of skills, and, finally, to an integrated and positive mutual exchange in their daily lives.

REFERENCE

Haley, J. Marriage therapy. *Archives of General Psychiatry*, 1963, *8*, 213–234.

CHAPTER 1

General Guidelines and Principles

This chapter provides an overview of the empirical and theoretical background and general guidelines for the social learning approach to marital therapy described in this manual. This bird's-eye view is important for two reasons. First, it provides a conceptual framework for understanding the various therapy techniques. Second, a grasp of the underlying theoretical principles, basic assumptions, and their empirical support will be helpful in guiding the therapist when unanticipated problems occur.

THEORETICAL AND EMPIRICAL BACKGROUND

Marital separation, divorce, and their aftereffects in the life events of the involved parties comprise a great stress on the psychological and physical functioning of individuals. Research on the stress produced by changes in lifestyle associated with separation and divorce—such as work and financial changes, change in residence and social activities, the loss of mutual friends, sexual problems, and the revision of personal habits—indicates that psychiatric and physical illness occur six to ten times more frequently for people with disrupted marriages (Bloom, 1975; Struening, Lehman, & Rabkin, 1970; Holmes & Masuda, 1973). Surveys of people who have sought professional help for psychological problems indicate that 42% of these individuals viewed the nature of their problems as marital and another 17% viewed their problems as pertaining to family relationships (Gurin, Veroff, & Feld, 1960).

Even when not followed by separation and/or divorce, marital distress and conflict are widely prevalent in our culture. There were 715,000 divorces in the United States in 1972, and it has been estimated that 40 million married couples need counseling (Kuhn, 1973).

Marital therapy of varied theoretical and clinical types has been practiced in the United States for nearly 50 years. However, until recently, there has been almost a complete absence of objective study and evaluation of marital therapy or marriage counseling. While proponents of the various "schools" of marital therapy continue to disparage the proponents of other schools, it is interesting to note that there are a number of common areas of focus in treating distressed marriages. For example, practitioners from divergent theoretical backgrounds tend to agree on the importance of clear communication between partners as a requisite for successful marriage (Ackerman, 1966; Lederer & Jackson, 1968; Satir, 1967; Gottman, Notarius, Gonso, & Markman, 1976).

Satir's functional communicator is able to do the following: he can ask for clarification if the message to him is unclear, ambiguous, or incongruent with the sender's thoughts or feelings; he can clarify and qualify messages he has sent that cause the receiver to ask for such clarification; he can ask for affective and cognitive feedback from the receiver of his messages; and he can give affective and cognitive feedback to the sender of messages that are congruent with his own feelings and thoughts. Similarly, Lederer and Jackson have emphasized the importance of clear communication, honesty, and trust in the marital system and provide a series of do-it-yourself practical exercises to aid their readers in developing these essential qualities. The social learning approach to marital therapy also views the establishment of good communication skills as an important therapeutic goal.

Lederer and Jackson have suggested that establishing a *quid pro quo* is essential in reorganizing a marriage. The behavior and attitudes of one partner always elicit some sort of reaction from the other. According to Lederer and Jackson, the therapist must analyze the repetitive, destructive patterns of interaction that regulate or rule the couple's relationship and help them establish new rules that are of mutual benefit. Similarly, in the social learning approach to marital therapy, spouses are trained to increase their recognition, initiation, and acknowledgment of pleasing interactions. From the social learning perspective, the couple's rules of interaction may be viewed as a *quid pro quo* system in which partners experiencing marital distress exchange a limited range and amount of reinforcement. One major goal of the social learning approach to marital conflict presented in this manual is to increase the level of reciprocity or mutually reinforcing exchanges between husband and wife. Patterson and Reid (1970) and Patterson and Hops (1972) have directly studied the reinforcement exchange systems in families and marriages. Their research identified two major patterns, *reciprocity* and *coercion*, as characteristic of distressed relationships.

Reciprocity refers to the equitable rates of positive reinforcement exchanged between partners. Reciprocal interaction between partners is characterized by their responsiveness to one another's requests and by their mutual reinforcement of each other's behavior. Thus, a wife's question, compliment, or request is acknowledged immediately; or a spouse's sexual advances are returned or postponed affectionately.

Coercion refers to interactions in which both partners engage in aversive actions that control the behavior of the other. Coercion can be observed when a request from one spouse takes the form of a strong demand. Noncompliance by the other spouse is punished by the escalation of aversive behaviors, such as criticism, withdrawal, or putdowns. Compliance by the intimidated spouse positively reinforces the demanding spouse's coercive style, and the spouse who "gives in" is negatively reinforced by a termination of the aversive demand. Patterson and Reid (1970) maintained that it is likely that if one partner uses coercion to control behavior, the other partner will also introduce this method of control. As Lederer and Jackson (1968) have phrased it, "Nastiness begets nastiness."

A SOCIAL LEARNING APPROACH TO MARITAL THERAPY

In the behavioral or social learning model are certain assumptions regarding what leads to satisfaction and what leads to dissatisfaction in a marriage. Maintaining marital satisfaction requires effort and commitment from both partners as well as the development of certain skills to ensure open and constructive communication. Marriage partners who are similar in their preferences, habits, and daily pace of life are likely to be companionable and happy together. However, the relationship between similarity and marital satisfaction is not as simple as the old cliché, "Likes attract." Rather, the concept of similarity embraces a wide variety of interactive styles and relationships. For example, in a happy relationship, spouses may be similar in their sleep–waking cycles and pace of life but different in their needs for socializing. Problems occur when differences occur in major areas of the relationship that outweigh the areas of similarity.

Each partner in a marriage has needs for affection, sex, recreation, companionship, approval, and status. In addition, each partner must contribute to the needs of the marital and family unit in the areas of finances, household chores and management, social activities, and child management. Satisfaction in marriage occurs as a result of *reciprocity* in providing for each of these individual and family needs. In other words, marital satisfaction results from the mutual exchange of words and actions that are pleasing to each spouse. Decades of research on human behavior indicate that the amount and range of pleasing actions that a partner *receives* are proportional to the amount and range of pleasing actions that he/she *gives.* This is the principle of reciprocity. You get what you give and you give what you get. When each partner is receiving an adequate amount of pleasing words and actions for his/her needs, the marriage will be experienced as satisfying to both spouses. Anger, disappointment, and frustration are a part of every relationship. However, when the exchange of negative feelings regularly exceeds the exchange of positive feelings, the result is discomfort, distress, and unhappiness with the relationship.

Marital dissatisfaction occurs when too few pleasing behaviors are exchanged between spouses, when pleasing interactions are limited to one area only (e.g., finances), or when one spouse gives many more "pleases" than he/she receives. This can happen when one or both spouses take pleasing behaviors for granted and ignore them; as a result, fewer pleasing actions occur as time goes on. Having one's needs go unmet often results in one or both spouses' using coercion, such as criticism, tantrums, nagging, threats, and violence. Coercive actions and words can be used to obtain one's needs rather than asking for pleasing events in an open and direct, but nonthreatening, manner. This brings us to the second assumption on which our marital counseling model is based: Increases in marital satisfaction will result when the spouses' ability to communicate both the positive and the negative aspects of their marriage is improved. It is the task of the therapist to teach couples communication skills that will increase their mutually rewarding exchanges, improve their ability to solve problems, and help their constructive expression of both positive and negative feelings.

The approach to marital counseling set forth in this book is primarily educational and aimed at producing change. It is designed to increase the skills of each partner in a marriage rather than to elicit insight why the marriage is floundering. This is not to say that insight by the spouses may not occur in the course of therapy. For us, insight is mainly a by-product of the couple's efforts to learn and use new communication skills to improve their relationship.

Because our emphasis is on helping couples to learn and apply new skills, the focus of therapy is on the present and working toward the future rather than on the past. For the couple the question is "Where do we go from here?" rather than dwelling on the whys and wherefores of past frustrations and unhappy events that cannot be undone. Since most spouses have a need to tell their side and vent the angry and hurt feelings from past events, they are given this opportunity in initial interviews with each spouse individually and with the couple. After the bad feelings are ventilated, recriminations about past wrongs are placed off limits and the couple is oriented to dealing with their relationship as it is now.

Since the goal of therapy is for the couple to learn new skills, the process you will employ as the therapist resembles active teaching or coaching rather than traditional therapy. As each skill is introduced to the couple, you will begin by giving a brief rationale on why the skill is important. Next, you will instruct the couple on how to use the skill. After you, as the therapist-"educator," have fully explained the skill, it is best to demonstrate both how to do it and how not to do it: "One picture is worth a thousand words."

For example, in the first session, you will be instructing the couple to become aware of and to acknowledge pleasing words and actions, or PLEASES. How *not* to acknowledge a PLEASE might be "I'm glad you took care of the kids this afternoon *for a change.*" "For a change" is a zinger that takes away from the positive acknowledgment of the PLEASE. Contrast this with "I really appreciate your taking care of the kids today." After the therapist has modeled *how not to* and *how to* express the feelings or ideas being taught, each spouse is asked, in turn, to practice or rehearse expressing the feelings or actions being focused on.

After they have tried it, you must provide feedback to them on how well they did. The feedback should be positive and specific, followed by suggestions for improvement, if necessary. Have them continue to rehearse the behavior or actions until each does it correctly. Preferably, the rehearsals should involve real situations that have occurred in the marriage. As the skills the therapist is teaching become more complex (e.g., negotiation) and deal with more emotionally charged issues (e.g., negative feelings), the amount of rehearsal needed will increase.

It may also be necessary for you to prompt or coach the spouse as he/she practices the skill. Prompting and coaching may involve gestures or signals on your part as the therapist indicating your approval, your wanting a spouse to slow down, to raise the level of his/her voice, or to keep eye contact with his/her partner. Coaching and prompting also involve giving verbal cues regarding the content of speech as each spouse tries to communicate his/her feelings. For example, as the therapist, you can prompt positive communication and assertion by saying, "Now make a positive request. What do you want your partner to do instead?" as the spouse is rehearsing the behavior. Prompting and coaching during rehearsal provide support and direction for spouses when they are trying a new skill that is difficult for them and/or expressing feelings they are not used to communicating. Remember to provide positive feedback after each rehearsal. Find something specific to compliment each time they practice; for example, eye contact, aspects of the content, or caring facial expressions. Adopt a "shaping" attitude, which means looking for and responding to small signs of improvement in the marital relationship. Remember that success will come with repeated practice of the skills. A shaping attitude on the part of the therapist is essential to the effectiveness of the therapy. Couples' success in learning the skills taught by this approach will come with repeated rehearsal followed by specific positive feedback for even small improvements. Each couple moves at its own pace through the behavior change process, some learning the skills quickly and easily and others struggling at each step.

Once the couple has practiced a skill successfully in the therapy session, homework assignments are given. The homework assignments ("Catch Your Spouse Doing Something Nice," executive sessions, and recreational activities) are the heart of the therapy process. One or two hours a week of therapy are not enough to change a relationship that is floundering. It is essential that the couple practice the skills in the home on a regular basis. Repeated practice in the natural environment will make the partners more comfortable in using their new skills. In this way, the effects of therapy can be extended and continued at home between sessions. We have found a strong connection between regularly completed homework assignments and the degree to which the couple's relationship improves. There are several things that you can do as a therapist to facilitate the couple's completion of homework assignments:

1. Stress their importance and explain how practicing at home can help.
2. Regularly review homework assignments and give time and attention to *completed* assignments rather than to why the couple did not complete assignments.
3. When the assignment is given after the couple have practiced a given behavior in the session, have them be specific as to when, where, and how often they will practice the skill at home.
4. Initially, it may be helpful for you or your secretary to call the couple during the week to see how the homework is coming. This acts as a reminder and also stresses the importance you place on their completing their homework.

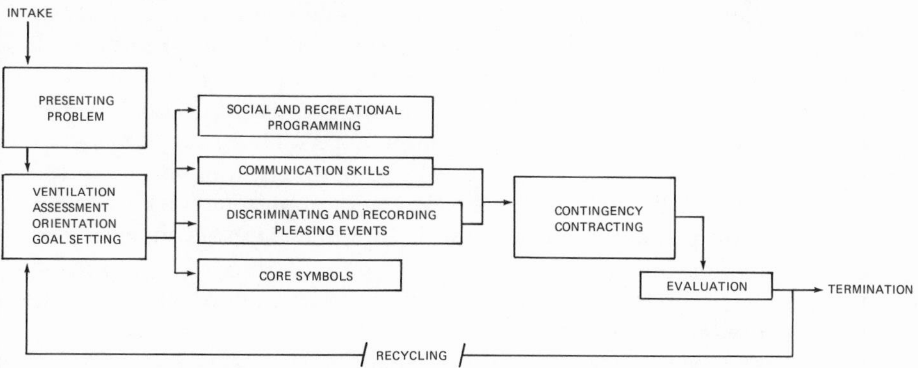

Figure 1. Flowchart of treatment modules in behavioral marital therapy. The initial sessions devoted to assessment, history taking, and ventilation of feelings should be done with a single couple. If marital therapy is to be done in a group setting, a group of three to five couples may be formed after these initial sessions and started at the social and recreational programming stages.

Figure 1 summarizes the process or flow of our therapeutic methods with married couples.

The sequence of the skills that are taught to couples in the therapy sessions is organized along two basic dimensions:

1. From simple to complex skills
2. From issues and content of a slow emotional tone and a focus on positives feelings to issues and content that have a high emotional tone and a focus on negative feelings

The reason for going from simple to complex is to build in success experiences by improving skills via small steps that can be easily mastered by the couple. We focus on neutral and positive topics initially for two main reasons. First, this focus helps the couple to begin to reorient their perceptions of each other and the marriage away from the negative toward recognizing the positive aspects of their relationship. Second, couples can learn new communication skills better if they start first with relatively nonthreatening issues. Once new skills are learned, they can begin to use them with a greater chance of success to communicate about issues and feelings that are more emotionally loaded.

THERAPEUTIC GOALS

By the end of therapy, a couple will hopefully possess the following behaviors:

1. They will understand the meaning and value of *reciprocity* as the exchange of positively valued actions and expressions in a relationship.
2. They will have increased the number, quality, and range of social, emotional, and instrumental behaviors that *please* their partners.
3. They will be more aware of and will more frequently acknowledge *pleasing* acts and words they receive from their respective partners.
4. They will be competent in verbal and nonverbal communication skills, which include:
   a. Giving PLEASES to the spouse
   b. Acknowledging PLEASES received from the spouse
   c. Requesting PLEASES (including physical affection) from the spouse in a direct, assertive manner
   d. Expressing *empathy* to the spouse by giving accurate feedback on what the spouse said and felt
   e. Expressing *negative* feelings and thoughts to the spouse in a direct, assertive, nonaccusative manner
   f. Requesting *pleasing* alternatives or termination of negatives in a direct, assertive manner
   g. Coping with unexpected hostility or "bad moods" by turning conversation toward mutually pleasing activities, giving repeated PLEASES in the face of hostility, taking time out, or giving *empathy*
5. A couple will have completed a *contingency contract* after suitable negotiation and compromise.
6. They will complete pre- and posttesting by filling out the Marital Adjustment Test. The responses from this questionnaire should demonstrate an improvement in marital satisfaction and a decrease in desires for change at the posttesting.

These goals, when attained, are the indications for a therapist's successful termination of the educational and therapeutic experience with a married couple.

CONDUCTING MARITAL THERAPY IN A GROUP

Marriage counseling in a group setting has been successfully implemented with a high degree of client satisfaction. Within each chapter, some special guidelines for working effectively in a group format are given in shaded blocks in the text.

What are the rationale and general guidelines for using behavioral marriage counseling in a therapy group, workshop, or class? There are advantages for both the therapist and the couples in using a group format for marriage counseling. For the therapist, the group format is cost-effective. It allows the therapist to see more couples in less time. This may be a particularly important consideration for therapists at mental health centers where too many clients and too few therapists make waiting lists necessary. With two marriage therapists running two short-term, 10- to 12-week groups concurrently, approximately 75 couples can receive marital therapy in a year. The same two therapists could offer similar types of individual or conjoint services to only 20 couples in the same period of time. From a cost-effectiveness standpoint, the groups could potentially generate fees of $15,000 (75 couples × 10 group sessions each = 750 service units at $20 per unit = $15,000), while the individual or conjoint services would generate only $8,000 in fees (20 couples × 10 conjoint sessions = 200 service units at $40 per unit = $8,000).

For the couple involved in marriage counseling, the group setting provides several advantages. First, in a group, there are more sources of feedback, more points of view, and more interchange and stimulation provided by other group members. Second, groups provide multiple models for various styles of interrelating as a couple. Exposure to different interaction patterns allows each couple a wide range of options to emulate, adapt, or avoid. Third, group feedback carries more impact and is often taken more seriously than feedback from a professional alone. Fourth, a group offers acceptance, support, and a safe learning environment as trust develops and couples discover that exploring their own relationship can be interesting and rewarding. Realizing that other couples also have severe problems and are able to make improvements in their relationships increases morale and therapeutic optimism. It has been our experience that the couples involved in group workshops usually ask for a reunion after the workshop is over, reflecting the amount of mutual support, cohesion, and *esprit de corps* that develops.

GUIDELINES FOR LEADING A MARITAL GROUP

If you are leading a therapy group, workshop, or class as a therapist or a counselor, you can selectively use your time and attention to reward those couples who are completing homework assignments. During homework review, couples who have completed their homework are encouraged to share the specific details of their experiences, giving a graphic recounting of the home experiences and providing an opportunity for group recognition of effort as well as of successes. Those couples who do not do their assignments are given less time rather than allowed a great deal of group attention to explore "why" they are not completing assignments. This sets a group norm that encourages effort, and this norm can have a powerful effect on recalcitrant group members. When reviewing homework, begin with a couple you think has been successful in completing the assignment. Then praise or "reinforce" the partners for whatever efforts or accomplishments their homework reflects. Selective attention to therapeutic work cues other couples to strive harder in a positive, nonthreatening way. Encourage feedback from other couples in the group by asking them what they thought was *good* about a completed assignment or a rehearsal of a new skill by one of the members or couples. This sets a norm for *positive* feedback. As the workshop leader, you can help in modeling *appropriate* feedback by being specific and by openly acknowledging the importance of specificity in the feedback coming from group members.

When teaching a new skill to the group, the therapist first models the skill and then asks one of the couples to try a rehearsal. It is best to begin with a couple who are likely to rehearse successfully, since this provides further opportunity for observational learning for couples who may have difficulty. Peer models are easier to identify with than the therapist, and therefore, the group offers greater potential for learning than does the conjoint therapy session.

The above guidelines for working with couples in a group format are general. More specific instructions regarding the adaptation of various counseling techniques to group therapy are presented in the chapters dealing with these techniques. The guidelines are set apart in the shaded blocks within each chapter.

REFERENCES

Ackerman, N. W. *Treating the troubled family*. New York: Basic, 1966.

Bloom, B. L. *Changing patterns of psychiatric care*. New York: Human Sciences, 1975.

Gottman, J., Notarius, C., Gonso, J., & Markman, H. *A couple's guide to communication*. Champaign, Ill.: Research, 1976.

Gurin, G., Verloff, J., and Feld, S. *Americans view their mental health. A nationwide interview survey*. New York: Basic, 1960.

Holmes, T. H., & Masuda, M. Life changes and illness susceptibility. In J. P. Scott (Ed.), *Separation and Depression*. Washington, D.C.: American Association for the Advancement of Science, No. 94, 1973, pp. 161–186.

Kuhn, J. R. *Marriage counseling: Fact or fallacy?* Hollywood, Calif.: Newcastle, 1973.

Lederer, W. J., & Jackson, D. D. *The mirages of marriage*. New York: Norton, 1968.

Patterson, G. R., & Hops, H. Coercion, a game for two: Intervention techniques for marital conflict. In R. E. Ulrich & P. Mountjoy (Eds.), *The experimental analysis of social behavior*. New York: Appleton-Century-Crofts, 1972.

Patterson, G. R., & Reid, J. B. Reciprocity and coercion: Two facets of social systems. In C. Neuringer & J. L. Michael (Eds.), *Behavior modification in clinical psychology*. New York: Appleton-Century-Crofts, 1970.

Satir, V. *Conjoint family therapy*. Palo Alto, Calif.: Science and Behavior Books, 1967.

Struening, E., Lehman, S., & Rabkin, J. Context and behavior: A social area study of New York City. In C. R. Wurster (Ed.), *Statistics in mental health programs*. Chevy Chase, Md.: National Institute of Mental Health, 1970.

CHAPTER 2

Getting Started

This chapter describes the tasks facing the therapist or counselor who is ready to start marital therapy or marriage counseling. Methods are suggested for all the specific steps involved in starting therapy, from recruiting clients to making a therapeutic contract.

RECRUITMENT AND REFERRALS

Recruitment of clients or patients for marital therapy consists of more than simply sending out announcements and distributing cards.

Personal contacts with referral sources are essential, using telephone calls, introductions, and direct conversations. To sustain a continuous stream of potential clients, you must also give follow-up information to professionals who refer people to you. Of course, all such information should only be provided with the client's signed permission.

Potential referral sources are legion. Lawyers—especially those who are willing to recommend counseling for clients who are filing for divorce—ministers, who feel that their parishioners need more than sympathy or advice, and doctors are among the more obvious. Schools need to know that they can refer families to you when the child may be the "identified patient" but the underlying problem lies in the relationship between the parents. Mental health clinics with waiting lists, marriage encounter groups and other marriage enrichment programs with couples who are too disturbed to benefit from their program, colleges with young marrieds or committed couples, private industry, social agencies such as Y's, rape centers, hot lines, suicide prevention centers, and programs for senior citizens should be explored as potential sources of referral. You might even want to work with police departments because of the constant calls they receive for help with domestic crises.

Satisfied ex-clients are usually the best referral source of all, and the experienced practitioner can look forward to and take pride in the building of this resource.

Good working relationships with doctors, psychiatrists, pediatricians, internists, ob–gyn specialists, and especially family and general practitioners can lead to referrals. Here is one way to encourage referrals systematically and to provide informational feedback to the referring agents. After sending an announcement card or letter describing you and your practice to the physicians in your area, call each physician's office. Don't insist on talking to the doctor; instead, ask the nurse or receptionist if you could stop by briefly sometime and leave some of your professional cards. Most will be polite and say yes. Within a week or so, go to the offices you have called and give some of your cards to the nurse or secretary. In most cases, they will offer to get the doctor to talk with you for a moment, if only for an introduction. Promise that you will not detain the doctor from his or her busy schedule and offer to come back again if it would be more convenient.

When the doctor comes out to meet you, be friendly, concise, and to the point in your salutation and introduction of yourself. Indicate clearly the kinds of services you provide and ask the doctor if he/she is getting satisfactory service from the mental health clinicians he/she is currently referring patients to. Say a few words about the distinctiveness of your services and practice. Assure the doctor that you are competent, have had many difficult cases before, and would provide feedback on the progress of patients referred to you. At the first indication of any disinterest, distraction, or impatience on the part of the physician, excuse yourself and leave. After the doctor refers a patient to you, immediately send that doctor a brief letter of acknowledgment, a preliminary evaluation, and a promise to send a progress report later. When you have completed the marital therapy, send the referring physician a brief treatment summary. If you follow these simple steps—prompting and reinforcing doctors for their referrals—you won't lack patients in your practice.

— • —

Mary had been referred by her family doctor when her headaches were not responding to prescribed treatments. The doctor suspected that her headaches had an emotional component that was possibly related to some marital problem. Mary had expressed some resentments toward her husband, Arthur, that the doctor felt were out of proportion to the situation. In the referring phone call, he was skeptical about the effectiveness of therapy and said his experience with "shrinks" had not been very satisfactory. He was reassured when we told him that we would remain in close contact with him and that we had seen couples with similar problems make improvements as a result of treatment. We gave an example of a case in which a wife's suppressed anger toward her husband took the form of acute colitis, which subsided after martial therapy. The doctor protested that Mary was able to express her anger too well, as their fighting often seemed to bring on her headaches. We explained that with help she could probably express her feelings more appropriately and less destructively. As a further step beyond headache relief and prevention, marital therapy might help Mary and Arthur get some pleasure from their marriage. The doctor seemed satisfied with this. After seeing the couple for the initial visit, we sent a note to the referring doctor thanking him for the referral and promising him a subsequent progress report.

— • —

Good working relationships with social workers, psychologists, and other counselors who do not specialize in marital therapy can lead to referrals, too. For example, informal consultations and conversations over coffee or lunch might lead to the realization that your colleague's patient(s) has an underlying marital problem. Children and adolescents with school and family problems are frequently reflecting marital dissension in the home. A thorough intake interview may reveal that marriage counseling is a more appropriate treatment than family therapy or direct work with the child or adolescent. Other examples of presenting problems that may seem unrelated to marriage problems are those where one partner in a marriage is referred for depression, anxiety, gynecological complaints, hysterical conversion symptoms, or psychosomatic symptoms. Even when both partners claim that the presenting problem is characteristic of the referred patient individually and that its onset preceded their relationship, it is well for you to educate your sources of referral to the fact that marital conflict and dissatisfaction may be exacerbating chronic or dormant symptoms. At the same time that you illustrate the situation in which marital therapy might be the treatment of choice, you might also help your referral source to convey to both partners why and how marital therapy would be beneficial to them. The referral agent may need help in order to "sell" his or her clients and patients on the idea that the problems are best treated in the context of their marital relationship.

Working well with referral sources involves close cooperation, prompt acknowledgment feedback, and follow-up. These measures should be pursued not only to increase your practice but also in the interest of sound professional and ethical relations.

INITIAL CONTACT

Warmth, sincerity, and accessibility can be communicated over the telephone to the patient even before the first visit. First impressions tend to set expectations, which, in turn, can powerfully affect outcome.

There should not be too long a wait for the first appointment—under a week if possible. The importance of the initial contact cannot be overemphasized, as it sets the tone for the ongoing relationship. If there is a receptionist or also other clerical persons involved in your

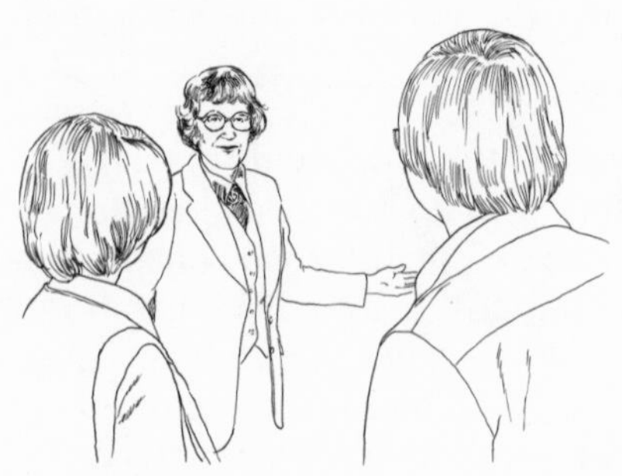

practice or clinic, in-service training should be undertaken for them. They need to be taught how to respond to questions such as, "What shall I do if my husband won't come in with me?" (answer: "You keep the appointment anyway and discuss it with the therapist"); "How much does it cost?" (answer: "$ _____ for the first visit, but why don't you discuss it with Mr./Ms./Dr._____ when you come in?"). They may need to be taught to be courteous, nonjudgmental, warm, and friendly and to exercise judgment of when to ask the therapist to call back immediately, as, for example, in cases of deep depression or if there is an indication of possible suicide or violence.

There are a number of ways in which you can make patients' first contact with you a pleasant and positive experience and thereby reduce anxiety and promote the early development of a therapeutic alliance. As a starter, you can give very careful directions for getting to your office or clinic. This can be done on the phone or by mailing a map with instructions for parking or public transportation. You might also check out with the couple whether they wish to be called by their first or last names and indicate how you would like them to call you. You should discuss and agree on fee arrangements with them before they leave the first session so that there is no confusion or misunderstanding about that sensitive topic. Some other routine, but helpful, transactions that can promote positive initial contacts are listed below:

1. Avoid having a desk as a barrier between you and the patients.
2. Give the patients a choice of where to sit, recognizing that some may want to be close to the door, especially during the initial contact.
3. Shake hands *after* the initial visit instead of at the opening introduction, as a handshake will mean more to the patients after they have come to know you a bit.
4. Use touching and "pats on the back" with discretion, taking into account the patients' comfort and values.
5. Greet the patients at the door to your office or in the waiting room, actively moving *toward* them at the start of a session.
6. Walk with patients to the door at the end of a session, saying "Goodbye" and reminding them of the next appointment, "I'll be looking forward to seeing you next week."
7. Apologize if you are late for an appointment.
8. Show patients where the toilet is located and give permission to use it whenever needed—even in the midst of a session.
9. Avoid looking at your clock or watch when the *patient is talking*.

INVOLVING THE RELUCTANT PARTNER

When only one partner appears for the initial interview or intake evaluation, you will want to convey the idea that, ideally, both partners should participate. Getting the reluctant spouse to enter therapy can be done in a number of ways. Never accept the assumption that an absent or reluctant husband or wife will not come in. Try to figure out the circumstances behind the absence or the reluctance, and help the willing spouse to deal with them. The first step is to find out how the presenting spouse has approached his/her partner so far regarding the need for treatment. Has the partner simply not been informed of the applicant's desire for therapy or counseling? Has it been with ultimatums? Has one partner threatened to file for divorce? Have you as the marriage counselor been set up as the "bad guy," as when one spouse tells another, "Wait until I tell the counselor about what you do!" You may find out that the absent partner was never invited to come to therapy or was never told about the appointment.

If the situation has been coercive, it may actually be helpful to train the present spouse to ask his/her partner in a positive, nonthreatening way to come in for at least one appointment. You might stress that you are not at all interested in assigning blame but rather in improving communication, that you will not be delving into the past but rather working on better ways of interacting in the present and future. It can also minimize the threat to explain that marital therapy or counseling is not the treatment of "sick" or "neurotic" people but an educational experience that aims at improving the relationship between husband and wife. You might point out that marital problems are influenced not solely by how neurotic either partner is (most people are neurotic to some degree) but by how each person's needs, interests, and personalities mesh or dovetail. The challenge of the initial evaluation process lies in establishing an accepting climate where each partner expects to explore and learn about the relationship in free give and take, rather than anticipating coercion, embarrassment and/or demands.

Whether or not the applying partner can approach the reluctant spouse in a skillful way regarding marriage counseling at this stage, you may wish to get in touch with the absent partner yourself by telephone or letter. Of course, you should first get the presenting spouse's permission to make this contact. If, as is usually the case, the reluctant partner is the husband, you can play by ear whether you want to invite him to give his side of the story, whether you want to stress how helpful it would be to you to learn what he can contribute to your understanding of the situation so that you can be more helpful to his wife, or whether you want to start off by issuing a direct invitation for him to attend a few evaluation sessions, after which you will make some recommendations to both him and his wife.

The important thing is to get the partner in. Sometimes the refusal to join is based on the belief that the marriage is virtually over and that there is no point in continuing. The reluctant spouse might say, "It's just no use" or "It just won't work." One way to counter this kind of discouragement is to suggest that the couple set a period of time within which they will make every effort, with professional help, to make the marriage as good as it can possibly be. Then, after a fair trial, they will know if it is either good enough or not. Without that extra effort, they will never know whether outside assistance might have helped the marriage to endure and become satisfying. This extra effort will also reduce the guilt felt by the partners if and when separation occurs.

If active solicitation of the reluctant spouse fails to involve the latter in treatment, the applicant should continue to come on his/her own. Pushing for dyadic participation in therapy is often in delicate balance, because if the therapist makes it mandatory rather than "ideal," the applicant may feel that there is nothing to be gained in coming alone and may lose an opportunity to learn ways of improving the marital relationship on his/her own or of getting help for him/herself. The other pitfall is to be so encouraging to the applicant to come in individually that not enough effort will be put into involving the reluctant partner.

ASSESSING MOTIVATION

The motivation for saving the marriage should be assessed. This can be done by asking each partner to rate desire to stay in the relationship and improve it on a scale of 0 (no desire, ready to split) to 10 (strongly committed to stay). Assessing motivation might be better addressed in a one-to-one format, since it can be devastating to a husband to hear that on a scale of 1 to 10, his wife pegs her motivation at 5 when he had assumed it to be a 9 or 10, and vice versa. It is useful information for you, however, because the higher the motivation, the more the individual is willing to make behavioral changes and the faster you can proceed in promoting changes.

Another item that is best taken up individually is whether or not there are outside liaisons. It is important to check this out early so that the possibility of game playing is ruled out. It does not help you to learn, after much work, that one partner has already planned to marry a lover and is going through counseling just to get the spouse "off his or her back." It is usually wise to get a commitment to fidelity—dropping any outside affairs—during the course of the treatments so that maximum effort is invested in improving the marriage. If a partner is unwilling to make such a commitment, the marriage is not likely to improve in the near future. You have several options to discuss with your client(s) at the point of finding resistance to giving up an outside liaison. One is to work with one or both partners individually, helping them to cope as well as possible with their personal and marital concerns. In this mode, you might help a partner develop independence and self-assertive skills in preparation for a possible rupture of the marriage. Assertion training sometimes has the effect of making this partner more attractive and desirable to his/her spouse and can lead to the latter's relinquishing the extramarital affair. Meanwhile, the partner who is immersed in an affair may be worked with individually to understand some of the unrealistic and disadvantageous aspects of the extramarital romantic attachment and thereby be helped to put his/her perspective in better balance.

Alternatively, you can see both partners together and have them focus on the positive and negative aspects of their relationship. This stock taking can sometimes help a partner who is involved in an affair to see more clearly what he/she stands to gain or lose by staying with or leaving the marriage. Even if your efforts to repair the marriage fail, the sessions will result in the clarification of personal goals and of the dissolution process without prolonging the double messages, confusion, pain, and doubt.

SEPARATION

You may be asked by one or both spouses if you feel a separation would help. Couples sometimes feel that a temporary separation will serve some vague, ill-defined purpose and may want to use it as a way of avoiding their problems or of delaying counseling. A visit, a rest, or a separate vacation for a change of scene can often be emotionally replenishing without risk of doing damage to the relationship, but separate residences are not to be recommended. Such an arrangement robs the partners of the opportunity to practice newly learned ways of interacting with each other. With separated partners, you would be attempting to do marriage counseling in a vacuum. Experience shows that such separations can lead to the exact opposite of what the couple is hoping for: a drop in motivation to build the marriage rather than a renewed determination to work on it. It can also result in an unintentional exploitation of the one left at home with all the responsibility, less income, and less companionship. With separations also comes the risk that one or both spouses will enter a new romantic entanglement that arouses excitement and diminishes the desire to expend efforts toward improving the old relationship. There is probably more risk of irreversibly damaging actions occurring during a separation than if they remain committed to working on their problems together.

If the couple inform you that they already have separated, the challenge is to plan for a new beginning. The key question is: How can their life be different when they get back together again? How can household tasks be reapportioned, finances rebudgeted, new mutual interests be generated, more physical and emotional space be provided? A new beginning must be maximized in every way with changes supported through carefully negotiated agreements. When the partner moves back into the home, the counseling should be intensified, as this represents a crucial period when, with help, the relationship can be sustained at a higher level of functioning. Without special effort and professional help, a reconciled couple can easily revert to the aversive communications that caused their separation in the first place.

CATHARSIS AND VENTILATION OF FEELINGS

During the evaluation sessions, you will want to become as knowledgeable as possible about the couple: prior backgrounds, parents' marriages, current attitudes and feelings. These early sessions, when therapist and patients are developing a trusting and special relationship, are the best time to encourage each partner to explore and ventilate her/his accumulated grievances, hurt feelings, anger, and recriminations. Catharsis, by allowing the person to get the bad feelings off his/her chest and feel better at least temporarily, will cement the therapeutic relationship. The partners will feel that you know all about their problems, have plumbed the depths of their emotional wounds and disappointments, and have a genuine concern for their total being.

You may want to meet with both partners first for an entire cathartic session, or you may want to break the sessions down into individual interviews and a couple interview. Each partner should have ample opportunity to express her/his resentments, and it is often better to do this without the other spouse present. This sort of "dumping" may be useful as a means of releasing and getting rid of hostility but should not be "laid on" the partner until it can be expressed in nondestructive ways, that is, until there has been some communication training so that it doesn't come across as an attack. Sufficient time must be allowed for ventilation so that the clients can get beyond the need to throw up the past and get on with the business of working on communication skills in the present. It will be next to impossible to set a ground rule on sticking to the present and the future and have it respected by the couple unless the positive work of therapy is preceded by sufficient time for shouting, tears, and breast-beating.

BUILDING FAVORABLE THERAPEUTIC EXPECTATIONS

In building realistically favorable expectations toward marital therapy, you can point out to the couple that you regard your goal not as preserving marriages or helping couples to endure conflict and unhappiness but as helping each spouse clarify and express his/her needs and desires so candidly and positively that it becomes eminently clear whether the required changes each must make are worth the effort. This approch gives each partner a view of what it will take to make the marriage work. Even if the therapy ends in divorce, partners are usually glad that they participated in marriage counseling because the clarifications and improved communication are so necessary for future decisions about what is best for the children, finances, community property, and other matters of mutual concern. After learning to communicate more openly and directly, mutual respect increases and there is less acrimony, vengefulness, blame, guilt, and bitterness. However, if there is any motivation at all for sticking with the marriage, and if the guidelines set forth in this book are followed, there is every reason to believe that the relationship can be improved to the point where both partners derive more joy from their marriage. Your conviction about this and the way you convey your optimism can do much to raise your clients' therapeutic expectations.

—— • ——

Anecdotes about similar couples with similar problems can also help to induce favorable expectations. For example, our prototypical couple, Mary and Arthur, were impressed by the story of a couple who were already separated when they came for marital therapy. The wife had filed for divorce, but her attorney had persuaded her to apply for treatment. She had agreed to come in for just one interview. She had been blaming her husband for her "nervous breakdown," and he was attempting to gain custody of their only child, based on the wife's "emotional instability." They became involved during the first session in developing an interim contract focused on ways that they could enjoy their son together and make plans for his future well-being. They had been concentrating so hard on mutual attack and blame that there had been no room for positive interaction. Starting with an area of shared interest, their child, they began a process that resulted in a much happier, stronger family unit than either had believed possible. Mary asked rather wistfully, "Do you think something like that could happen to us?"

— • —

Revealing humorous anecdotes about incidents in marital therapy can allay apprehensions and promote positive attitudes in the first few sessions. Couples may dread counseling because it seems so threatening and ominous, and to hear that part of it is fun can alleviate some of these fears. Arthur was particularly amused when we told him about a previous couple who took their homework exercises on communication too seriously. The wife in this case called up and asked the therapist if she and her husband were allowed to communicate at other times or only when the homework assignments on communication were to take place. Her husband was saying that he wasn't supposed to listen to her the rest of the time!

A few quoted positive statements from "graduates" can also contribute to an optimistic attitude. We told Mary and Arthur about another couple who said, two years after successfully completing marital therapy, that their third and fourth honeymoons were so much better than their first. Their child, who had stopped having nightmares, asked how come they weren't fighting anymore. You may want to provide words of encouragement about how much the couple have going for them, stressing whatever mutual values or strengths have emerged from the evaluation sessions. For instance, they can be reminded that they have managed to stay together for X number of years, that they share equal concern for their children (if they do), and that they both have made a giant step toward the resolution of their difficulties just by being with you in your office. This reflects a new situation that can represent a new beginning for them. Each can take comfort in the fact that his/her partner does care enough to make this significant step of engaging in marital therapy. If one or both partners say that they have had counseling before that did not work, you can respond affirmatively that the present therapy will be of a different form and can be the beginning of a new phase in their marriage.

A handout, such as "An Introduction to Marital Therapy," located in the "Client's Workbook," can also be an effective device for developing positive therapeutic expectations. If you are in an agency or clinic, you may want to get a committee together to write a brochure that applies to your particular setting and brand of marriage counseling. If you are in private practice, you will want to design a similar statement that is adapted to what you have to offer. Use it as a tool to elicit more questions and other reactions from therapy applicants so you can discover "where they are coming from" and involve them actively in therapy from the start. In this way, you can start addressing their immediate concerns and avoid resorting to lecturing. A handout can be used as points of departure for giving the couple a clear idea of what happens during therapy. It structures realistically favorable expectations and reduces anxiety over the unknown.

If a marital partner has been making unrealistic demands of the other partner and is now looking toward marriage counseling as a means of "making" the spouse "see the light" and change in desired directions so that they will "live happily ever after," then it is important that this misguided enthusiasm be tempered with perspective. Perhaps some romantic illusions are getting in the way of realistic expectations. You may have to help one or both spouses to consider imposing certain painful but realistic limits on the potential of the marriage. Realistic potential for change should be mutually assessed, with you as the therapist serving as a mediator, to form a solid basis for goal setting. For example, the fact that Leon was confined to a wheelchair with a progressive, terminal disease meant a scaling down of his and his wife Ruth's expectations of the treatment. But they were helped to get the very most out of the time they had left together once they accepted more limited goals. Large numbers of children or childlessness, dependent grandparents, physical or mental limitations, financial constraints, educational or vocational handicaps, and major differences in background and personality should be noted as therapeutic expectations are shaped. Therapeutic expectations should be based on:

1. A realistic anticipation of the possible changes that can be made based on awareness of limitations as well as potentialities
2. A positive outlook toward improving the marriage with full regard for potentialities in spite of the limitations

Your attitude, expressed both verbally and nonverbally to your patients, is the key to setting the expectations. The fact that you are looking forward to working with them and feel that it will be challenging, worthwhile, and fun is all-important and should be communicated with words, tone of voice, gestures, and facial expression.

The positive changes that often take place after just one interview are surprising and rewarding for both therapist and clients. There is often a surge of hope and a sudden renewal of tenderness. It is hard to know how much of this is due to each partner's willingness to try working on the relationship and how much is due to what actually transpires during the interview. Of course, you want to capitalize on this "honeymoon effect" by reinforcing it and translating it into positive therapeutic expectations.

ESTABLISHING A POSITIVE THERAPEUTIC RELATIONSHIP

The importance of developing a close, trusting relationship with both partners cannot be overemphasized. The therapeutic relationship with both husband and wife is the supporting structure and conduit for the specific techniques that will be described in later chapters. If it is necessary to see one partner more than the other, it is important that both of them feel your emotional support and understanding equally. If there should be less rapport with one partner, this must be dealt with by allowing equal time, by discussing it openly, or by providing a balance in some other way. Sometimes, it can be therapeutic to involve a second therapist. For example, let us suppose that you are a woman therapist and that you have a client in a women's assertiveness-training group. She finally develops enough skill to persuade her husband to apply with her for marriage counseling, but there are indications that he would find it difficult to confide in a woman, and particularly in you, since he knows you have a prior relationship with his wife. It might be appropriate to invite a male therapist or counselor to join you for the intake or evaluation interview. The husband might need to be seen individually or in a group to provide the balance needed to help him become equally involved. These balancing arrangements can help avoid his seeing you as "belonging" to his wife or his feeling that there are two women "against" one man. Involving a co-therapist is expensive and not often necessary, but it can be useful in situations where resistance derives from difficulties in relating to a therapist of the opposite sex. Co-therapy can also be useful for training purposes and for modeling effective man–woman communications for the couple(s).

THE MARITAL HISTORY AND RELATIONSHIP INVENTORY

In taking a complete and interactional history, which is part of the evaluation process, the therapist solicits information about past influences on the marriage and current resources for change as viewed by each partner:

1. *Parental and cultural background.* Each partner brings to the marriage a set of role expectations that are the result of his/her

accumulated previous experiences, cultural background and norms, and parental models.

2. *Patterns of interaction.* Marital therapy starts with the couple's habits, dynamics, and distribution of social interaction in major areas of married life, such as children, sex, affection, chores, finances, recreation, and decision making.
3. *Tuning in to each other: Who wants what from whom?* The prognosis of the marriage will depend in part on each partner's ability to develop awareness of and concern for the needs and desires of the other.

These elements cannot be separated in actual practice, and they are being continually assessed throughout treatment even after the formal evaluation period is over. As you explore past experiences, relevant linkages to their present patterns of interaction will occur to the couple. Questioning your clients about their own and their partner's needs will begin to broaden the focus of their thinking about what they had in the past that was good.

PARENTAL AND CULTURAL BACKGROUND

It can be helpful for you to know how each partner recollects and feels about his/her respective parents' roles. The parental role models that are of significance are not necessarily his/her parents. A client may be identifying more closely with a grandparent, a stepparent, a fosterparent, an adoptive parent, a friend's parent, a surrogate parent, or even a fantasy parent. Often without awareness, clients make efforts to turn their marriage into a carbon copy of their parent's marriage or, in the case of negative attitudes toward their parents' marriage, the opposite. For example, Rex had witnessed such bitter conflict between his parents that when his wife, Estelle, presented him with an argument, no matter how mildly, Rex withdrew in panic for fear that it would develop into the kind of brawling that he had been exposed to as a child. One reason for Arthur's limited tolerance of Mary's headaches was that he associated them with his mother's use of her heart condition to control his father.

If a client's parents were divorced, that fact can engender an overreaction in one of two directions. He/she may be terrified of divorce or, on the other hand, may have a tendency to turn to divorce too readily as the easy way out when confronted with minor difficulties. The type of reaction depends on the subjective experiences and actual consequences generated by the parental divorce.

Husbands and wives have actual and idealized roles in the areas of responsibility, affection, and power that are derived from their childhood experiences. These role expectations involve concrete behaviors, such as who does the gardening, who initiates sex and affection, who handles the money, who takes out the garbage, who reads to the children, who drives the car, how often conversations are held, and who answers the telephone. In contrast to overt role behaviors and expectations, the intangible, nonverbally expressed concern over affection, tasks, and authority is even more pervasive, though more subtle.

—— • ——

Oscar and Penny were a couple to whom the importance of who took care of the firewood for their fireplace had become a major issue. It symbolized all of their role expectations. Oscar had been brought up to believe that it was emasculating to do household chores, and he also felt that it was beneath his dignity as a clergyman to be concerned with such "mundane matters." Penny had been raised in a complementary manner; that is, she had submissively assumed the role of household drudge in accord with her observational learning of her parents' interaction. When it became too much for her, Penny went to the other extreme, aggressively demanding that Oscar suddenly bear more than his share of the burdens to make up for her having done more than her share for so long. It took many weeks of marital therapy for them to reach a balanced, collaborative, teamwork approach to sharing the household responsibilities. No real progress could be made until they were helped to take a good hard look at what had shaped their attitudes in the past. This involved inviting both of them to share family background information. The aloofness of Oscar's father (who was a bishop), his detachment from his family, his putting the needs of his parishioners ahead of the needs of his wife and children were brought out and put into perspective.

—— • ——

Cultural factors are basic to role expectations for men and women, children and adults, and parents and grandparents. For example, from our experience working with couples of Mexican extraction, it may be asking too much of a traditional Mexican male to accept marriage counseling from an Anglo female or to accept the idea of his wife's seeing a male therapist in a one-to-one counseling situation. Working with Mexican-American couples is another situation where co-therapists can perform a useful function in bridging gaps in understanding due to cultural differences. We have found it helpful for a female therapist to initially work individually with the Mexican wife while a male therapist sees the husband. After two to five separate sessions, during which time trust builds and acceptance of exploration and change grows, the couple is often ready to pursue marital therapy conjointly or in an ethnically compatible group. If one or both therapists can speak the clients' language, both literally and figuratively, it can be supportive to the couple and cut down on the number of dropouts. Sharing the basic language of your clients also may be helpful in uncovering subcultural barriers to the communication between the partners. Without a knowledge of the clients' ethnic traditions, it is easy to make insensitive suggestions regarding interactions with in-laws, the subject of women working, the discipline of children, sexual practices, holiday rituals, and many other emotionally charged areas. Some minority couples assume so much responsibility for relatives that it puts stress on their marital relationship. But if this concern for the extended family represents a deeply felt obligation held by either or both partners, it must be discussed within the context of the clients' value system.

There is a cultural foundation underlying sexual attitudes and behaviors. Screening for sexual problems is done by exploring attitudes about sex stemming from past experiences, as well as focusing on sexual interaction in the present. It is usually necessary to do some exploration with the partners of how sexual information was first conveyed to them. At what ages did they learn about sex, from whom, and with what emotional overlay? If there were strong taboos and a great deal of guilt induction, a thorough review of the impact on the client with considerable interpretation and support may be necessary.

Sexual problems resulting from guilt about childhood experimentation or traumatic experiences, such as molestation or rape, have to be shared and understood before they can be dealt with therapeutically. It can be helpful to know what sex was like for the client prior to marriage or during previous marriages and also if there have been any changes in the frequency and level of satisfaction from the earlier stages of this marriage. What changes in other aspects of their lives preceded or were associated with the changes in their sexual communication? A skillfully taken history and an interview can do much by themselves to demystify and desensitize sexual hang-ups and misconceptions. By *skillful,* we mean direct, nonjudgmental, supportive questioning, using terms that are not too scientific to be understood. To direct your treatment efforts efficiently toward the critically important problem areas requires a thorough understanding of the couple's pattern of interaction. For any particular distressed marriage that you are evaluating, you will undoubtedly uncover several maladaptive and recurring patterns of interrelationships.

PATTERNS OF INTERACTION

A rich source of knowledge about the interactional patterns in marriage comes from a couple's behavior as you directly observe it. Notice who tells his/her story first and how the other reacts. Be alert to how disagreement is expressed. As they respond to your questions, take note of how value conflicts are described. Do they listen to each other? Is the communication direct or are there double messages, hidden agendas, or scapegoating? Does one spouse tend to be aggressive, thereby inviting passivity in the other? Does there appear to be a top dog–underdog relationship? How is decision-making power shared? Has there been violence or is there a subtle type of exploitation going on? If so, how is it provoked or reinforced by the victim? What are the threats? What are the strengths in the relationship? Do the partners sit close to each other? Do they touch each other or smile at each other? Are there flashes of mutual understanding and intimacy? By careful probing and sensitive observation of verbal and nonverbal interaction, you can begin to identify patterns of interaction that are important reflections of what actually occurs in the home. From these observations, you can assess the behavioral assets as well as the deficits in each partner and in the relationship.

The "Marital Pre-Counseling Inventory" (Stuart & Stuart, 1973) provides a framework for a family time-study of a couple's daily routine. This is a useful and comprehensive assessment device that is recommended as a means of obtaining important information about each of the spouses and their relationship. It takes a person about an hour to complete the inventory, and you will have to assist clients with less than a high school education to fill it out. Each partner completes an Inventory, and you can evaluate the understanding of each other's attitudes and feelings by comparing their respective responses.

Another way to obtain this kind of information is to have the clients keep their own daily log. You, the therapist, and they, the clients, can get a picture of when fights or togetherness and lovemaking usually occur, along with what precedes and what follows. The so-called out-of-the-blue blowups can have antecedent and consequent determinants that belie their presumed spontaneity. The headaches that allegedly have "nothing to do with the marriage" should be assessed in the context of the marital events and interactions that precede and follow them to identify possible precipitants and secondary gains or payoffs. Many times the connections between the emotional, behavioral, and psychosomatic problems and their environmental antecedents and consequences are not obvious to the couple and demand scrutiny by the therapist.

Mary's headaches invariably occurred when Arthur was home. She seemed amazed to hear herself say, "I can't afford to have a headache when there's no one to watch Lisa." Out of the careful questioning during the evaluation sessions came the implication and insight that the headaches might be under her voluntary control, or at least more subject to environmental stimuli than she had realized.

If the couple are staying together through threats of punishment or aversive control, this needs to be brought out early in the interviews. For example, a husband might be controlling his wife by threatening to withhold money, or a wife might be controlling her husband by threatening to leave him. At times, coercive elements in the relationship can be subtle; for example, in some distressed marriages a partner may become cheerful and open to conversation only when his/her demands or expectations are met by the other.

There are other maladaptive patterns of marital interaction that can be identified during the initial evaluation sessions. A typical problem involves relationships characterized by an insufficient exchange of reinforcement or PLEASES, or a situation in which more PLEASES are given by one partner than are received. This is usually felt as "being taken for granted" by the partner who is not getting enough recognition.

Sometimes provocative, negative behaviors become reinforced or ingrained because they produce emotional reactions in the spouse; for example, the wife shouts at the husband for his passivity, and he responds by sulking and cursing to himself, while his increased passivity arouses her anger. His passivity is reinforced by her shouting and her shouting is reinforced by his cursing. Any behavior that generates strong emotional reaction—positive or negative—in a loved one tends to be powerfully reinforced.

Other maladaptive interactional patterns that are found in unhappy marriages might include putting each other down, ignoring each other or withdrawing from contact with each other, and looking outside of the marriage to satisfy one's needs.

The internal biorhythms of the partners can often be at variance, thereby producing conflicts and dissatisfactions. When a "day person" marries a "night person," problems of synchronization can occur. An early riser who gets sleepy by 9:00 P.M. has a hard time keeping up with a spouse who likes to sleep late in the morning and carouse until dawn. Partners can have different preferences regarding the time for making love and may need help making compromises in their sexual communication.

A daily or hourly log of how each of the spouses feels about their ongoing activities can be useful in pointing out the crucial times of day or periods when tensions build and attempts at discussion are more likely to erupt into arguments. In some families, there are hassles every morning in getting the children off to school and the adults off to work. In many families, the interval between Daddy's coming home and dinner is fraught with bickering. The daily log can pinpoint the times and situations that are high-risk for conflict and lay the basis for effective negotiations later. Providing time and space to unwind, cutting the cocktail hour short, and postponing discussion of sore subjects until later are acceptable alternative strategies for couples who get insight into their maladaptive patterns of interaction from their own daily logs. Many have come to realize the pitfalls of arguing on an empty stomach.

—— • ——

Maggie agreed to take her two small children for a walk around the block every night that Walter came directly home from work. This chore was worth it to her when she realized that his being met at the door by demands for attention had led to his unwinding at a bar instead of at home. Providing Walter space and quiet for those few minutes changed the climate at their home. There was less tension at dinner, and Walter learned to relate to the children more positively. He was ready to play with them and read to them after dinner in a way that he simply could not manage without a transition from a pressured day at work.

—— • ——

The most common areas of marital disharmony are finances, child management, use of leisure and social time, distribution of household chores, relatives, affection and sex, and communication in general. Communication can be conceptualized as existing on three different levels: verbal, affectional, and sexual. As verbal communication improves, the other two levels often fall into place. With a decrease in resentments in other areas, there is more chance for a breakthrough in the barriers to sexual communication.

Sometimes the conflicts are embedded in different value systems. For example, basic philosophical differences in child rearing may be hard to negotiate and may need ancillary approaches, such as a parent training workshop, to help the partners get together on a mutual approach to discipline. Conflicting values, preferences, and moral stances on sexual matters can be complex and often need to be thoroughly explored. In-law problems, too, can be difficult to work out because of family ties based on dependency, respect, or loyalty to parents. One spouse may value close ties to other relatives far more than the other spouse. We have been impressed by the dramatic results that have been achieved between couples and relatives as a result of rather simple interventions, such as direct instruction or assertion training. One intervention was recommending strongly that less time be spent with in-laws. Another was having a couple communicate their appreciation of their parents' concern for them but firmly indicating that they would make their own decisions and would not tolerate their partner's being bad-mouthed by relatives.

With all these areas of conflict and interaction, it is how the partners are relating to each other that needs to be recognized and incorporated into the marital history and Inventory. Are the children being used as pawns or being asked to take sides? Is money being used to establish power, or is sex being used as a weapon? What are the fight patterns? Who gives in? How are arguments resolved? Is the anger internalized so that there is gunnysacking, depression, or martyrdom? Are there relationships such as the spendthrift and the miser; wife as dutiful child and husband as parent, or vice versa; or "indulgent parent" and "strict parent to compensate"? What games are being played? What is the emotional economy that keeps the marriage in balance, and what has shaken this balance to the point where one or both are asking for help now? What triggered help seeking *now,* at this particular point in time? What does each partner expect or hope to get from you and the marital therapy? The two-way or reciprocal nature of the couple's interactions is what you need to grasp at the outset so that your interventions can be on target.

TUNING IN TO EACH OTHER: WHO WANTS WHAT FROM WHOM?

Accurate assessment of each partner's capacity for empathy during the initial evaluation results in two gains. First, it establishes each partner's baseline of ability to tune in and understand his/her spouse's feelings and attitudes. Second, it promotes a higher level of awareness and concern for one another's thoughts and feelings; thus, the assessment process leads very naturally into treatment.

There are several efficient ways of assessing the empathy of the partners. The willingness of one person to engage in recreational pursuits of the other partner's choosing is a telling barometer of levels of empathy. The extent to which the partners back each other up in the disciplining of their children or support each other in the presence of other people is also a clue.

In the sexual area, it is important not only to learn the frequency of intercourse and who initiates it but also how each partner feels about this pattern. Find out whether they can ask for changes that they want in their lovemaking. Can they respond to their partner's requests for changes, or do fear of rejection, feelings of being threatened, or defensiveness interfere with this sort of communication? Often it is the wife who wants more verbal and affectional communication, while the husband is asking for more sexual responsiveness and variation. Turning points sometimes occur when a husband in this kind of a situation agrees to more romantic verbal interchange than he feels completely comfortable with or when a wife agrees to initiate sex in spite of her shyness.

There are "diagnostic games" that can be utilized in early interviews to evaluate empathy and promote mutual involvement at the same time. These exercises can be the first step in teaching spouses to be specific in framing their likes and dislikes, to be aware of their wants, and to be able to put their requests in specific terms. To shape specificity and more positive requests, you may want to have each partner say to the other, "I like it when you . . . because it makes me feel . . ." A simple exercise like this one can be used repeatedly in the treatment process for building communication skills that enhance the capacity to empathize, compromise, negotiate, and finally to contract.

Have both partners identify positive resources and assets in the other person, even if it means going back to why they married the spouse in the first place. For example, if each feels that the other is a good parent, this can mean that there is a relatively favorable prognosis for the marriage. Another "opener" during the evaluation process is to ask a wife to identify a need of her husband and to tell what more she would be willing to do to help meet that need, and vice versa. This can result in some poignant reappraisals of how they have been interacting and what personal investments they would be willing to make to improve their marriage.

Another diagnostic game is to ask each partner to name three things his/her partner likes about him/her and three things he/she does not like. Then have each partner check out the accuracy of these predictions. Sometimes all six items are correct. For example: "He likes my cooking, the way I dress, and the way I treat his parents, but he hates the way I nag, yell at the children, and resist entertaining." "She likes my looks, the way I make love, and the way I provide for the family, but she hates the way I refuse to help around the house, work late without telephoning, and procrastinate about taking her out." If these responses are all on target, it affords you the opportunity to point out that their communication is not all that bad since, at least, they each know where the other is coming from. On the other hand, if this exercise leads to responses like, "There isn't anything she likes about me" or "It's not the messy house that bugs me—for fifteen years I have been trying to get across to you that it's the sulky way you greet me when I come home from work that gets me down," this tells you, and them, something, too.

Questionnaires filled out by the couple can help in assessing current and potential areas of empathy. One is the "Areas of Change" questionnaire (Weiss, Hops, & Patterson, 1973), which reveals not only what each partner wants of the other but also what each feels would please the other. This is a further step toward helping each to decide what he/she is willing to invest in improving the marriage by attempting to meet the needs of the other. This questionnaire is particularly illuminating because of the specificity of the behaviors listed and the emphasis on desired frequency of these behaviors. There are 34 specified behaviors falling into categories such as household chores, appearance, social life, sex, child care, and use of leisure time. The "Areas of Change" questionnaire can be obtained by writing to Robert Weiss, Ph.D., Department of Psychology, University of Oregon, Eugene, Oregon 97403. Another particularly comprehensive questionnaire is the "Marital Pre-Counseling Inventory" (Stuart & Stuart, 1973), which was mentioned in the last section. It gives in-depth assessment of empathy by asking each spouse to estimate the feelings and attitudes expressed by the other in various areas of marital life. The degree of agreement and mutual understanding or misunderstanding can be ascertained and used for targeting treatment goals and measuring treatment progress and outcome.

With Mary and Arthur Peabody, more social and personal history was obtained from Mary than from Arthur, as she was only too willing to describe her mixed-up childhood struggle for an education. Arthur was more reticent in discussing his past. Mary contrasted the lack of support she had experienced from her parents with the overinvolvement of Arthur's mother in their affairs. She said, "Arthur's mother spoiled him and now he expects too much from me. It's just not fair!" It became quickly obvious that different role expectations were part of the problem and, although more background information would be useful, it was important at this point to help them focus on how their relationship could be improved in the present rather than getting stuck in the past. Exploration of Arthur's relationship with his mother could be deferred, but Mary had to be stopped from "diagnosing" Arthur's problems and trying to ally herself with the therapists in treating him as the patient. Moving away from labeling and from the why's to "what can we do to make things better" was the sounder approach. It was a case of moving from recriminations to renewal of hope.

When they were seen individually, they were asked about their motivation for continuing the marriage. In spite of Mary's more verbal complaints, Arthur rated his motivation, on a scale of 1 to 10, as only at point 5, while Mary felt she was somewhere between a 6 and a 7. This indicated that Mary might have to make more effort than Arthur, at least initially.

It is understandable that Arthur raised many questions about fees. His professional orientation, as well as his feelings of insecurity in relation to their financial situation, was reflected in the concern he expressed over the amount of $40 per hour. He was relieved to hear that the expected course of treatment was not more than approximately three months and that he could pay for it over a longer period of time than that, if necessary. It became clear that their attitudes about money were different and that they used this difference as a focal point for some of their hostility, so getting amicable agreement on the fee was an important first step. It was also an early learning experience for them in negotiating and clarifying a sensitive issue.

THERAPEUTIC GOALS

Goals should be realistic and shared and derive naturally from the assessment process. While the setting of goals is an important phase in the early stages of therapy, it requires continued vigilance and possible revision throughout the entire period of treatment or counseling. If one partner anticipates gaining more power at the expense of the other, or if one spouse has excessively high expectations of the other's ability to change, there need to be clarification, negotiation, and compromise. There may need to be some clarification of conflicting values, or some scaling down of romantic expectations of what marriage is really like. Goals may be set for changes in any of the areas of marriage: child management, finances, recreation, sex, and conversation. Succeeding chapters will illustrate the range of goals that may be set. Goals should be specific, positive, and functional and should have a high likelihood of success. Functional goals are interactions or activities that are likely to occur frequently in the couple's life together and that can provide natural sources of satisfaction and pleasure. For example, with a couple that is withdrawn and noncommunicative, it is more functional to help them work on end-of-the-day greetings than on how to acknowledge each other's birthdays more affectionately. Birthdays occur only once a year, but seeing each other after work is a daily event and can be a richer source of affectionate exchanges. It is important that you not impose your values on the goals formulated by the spouses, although it may be advisable to state openly your biases and preferences as they relate to the form and quality of marriage, and that you move one step at a time, generating hope and confidence in the work that lies ahead.

THE THERAPEUTIC CONTRACT

The contract between you and the couple represents the culmination of the evaluation process. It specifies what the therapist can provide and, in exchange, what the clients are expected to give in terms of fees, attendance, length of treatment, confidentiality, and treatment objectives. This contract is not to be confused with the contingency contract between the husband and wife, which is dealt with later in Chapter 6. The purpose of the contract between therapist and clients is to clarify and specify mutual expectations and to affirm mutual commitment regarding treatment. The word *commitment* is defined as a promise or pledge to do something and also as an act of doing or performing something, and the process of developing the contract should encompass both definitions. It can demonstrate that each spouse can, with adequate reinforcement, respond to positive expectations.

A sound therapeutic contract protects the rights of the clients to receive counseling from qualified therapists, so it should include your credentials. Treatment goals should be mutually set, understood, and agreed upon. They are subject to revision, as they are not static, but the revisions should be jointly made (Stuart, 1975). There should be descriptions of the treatment procedures in nontechnical language and indications of what the clients may expect to experience during the course of treatment. Any side effects or risks involved in the treatment should also be pointed out.

Fees, of course, should be specified in advance. Financial arrangements must be precisely formulated for ethical as well as therapeutic considerations. This holds true whether you are operating in the public or in the private sector. If you have a sliding scale, be sure that it is consistent and that you avoid any appearance of collusion with clients versus insurance companies by putting a disproportionate number of insured clients at the higher end of the scale. The fee must be understood at the outset because later misunderstanding can have disastrous results, such as feeding resistance or causing premature withdrawal from treatment. In situations where no fee is charged, such as in community mental health centers, where married couples' groups are established as an educational service, it is wise to institute a contingency, "good faith" deposit returnable for attendance. The couples may be asked to submit a $10–20 deposit, increments of which are returned to them at each session they attend of the ten-session workshop. This incentive to attend regularly often works well. In our experience at the Oxnard (California) Community Mental Health Center, consistent attendance at educational workshops for married couples rose from 40% to 80% with institution of the contingency deposit.

The agreements about time also have serious ethical components, since both therapists and clients tend to work harder if treatment is time-limited as opposed to being open-ended. Mutual understanding regarding goals, fees, and time expectations prevents endless, ill-planned treatment, which is unfair to all concerned. You may want to build in ways of providing for extensions after certain defined time periods have elapsed, based on evaluations of progress. It may be a relief to a reluctant partner to have three sessions suggested with the understanding that there will be a mutual reassessment at that point. The next time block might include a couples' group, some individual sessions, or supplementary therapy of another kind to cover another set number of weeks. The planning for definite time sequences should be individualized. For example, therapy can be scheduled for X number of sessions, until the baby is born, until the husband has to go out to sea again, until the wife returns to night school, or until they leave on the trip to celebrate their 10th wedding anniversary. Sequential planning sets goals in a framework that can provide incentives and make it easier to review and reinforce progress. Having a time structure also helps the couple anticipate the termination from the start, thereby enabling appropriate expectations and realistic concerns to balance the fears about ending.

As in all other phases of life, awareness of an ending point has an antiprocrastination effect. The time-limited therapy model acts as a spur to making maximum use of intervening opportunities. Then, if reassessment results in a plan for further treatment, all the advantages of a new beginning can be maximized in a way that ongoing treatment without these meaningful intervals, breaks, or reevaluation points would not provide. Frequency of sessions, length of sessions, duration of therapy period, and availability of the therapist in between sessions should be worked out in advance. Other relevant questions to be covered are whether telephone calls are acceptable, whether calling you at home is acceptable and under what circumstances, and whether or not fees will be charged for telephone conversations or for broken appointments.

The time involved in carrying out homework assignments is another factor that should be discussed. The couple have a right to foreknowledge about the extent of the investment that will be required of them in terms of time as well as money. Homework, or *instigation therapy,* as it is sometimes called, is an essential part of marriage counseling. One or two hours a week with you in a clinic or office is inadequate unless something happens during the other one hundred and sixty-six or sixty-seven hours of the week. The content of the homework assignments will be suggested throughout this book. Some weeks, homework will involve planning and carrying out recreational activities, while at other times it will involve communication exercises. Thus, the initial contract should include at least the clients' verbal voluntary commitment to accept and follow through on reasonable homework assignments to the best of their ability. Learning is most effective when it is voluntary, and the more dedication is put into the learning exercises, the more likely that gains will be made.

Examples of contracts that include individualized items are agreements that involve attendance at Alcoholics Anonymous meetings during the course of treatment, the use of prescribed psychoactive medication (especially in cases where a spouse has well-documented schizophrenia or manic–depressive illness), or limitations on time spent with interfering in-laws or with single friends who evoke jealousy in a partner. You might want to build in a clause to ensure a supplementary service, such as participation in a parents' workshop, if child management is one of the couple's areas of conflict.

Other important client rights to be borne in mind are the right to refuse treatment or to end treatment and the rights of privacy and confidentiality.

The degree of formality of the contract is dependent on your own and your clients' discretion and preferences. You can institute "legalistic" procedures, such as witnessed signatures, or you can keep it anecdotal and simple. However, basic items that should always be included pertain to (1) goals, (2) fees, (3) time frames, and (4) homework assignments. Remember that the contract is a two-way interaction and that your clients need to know what they can expect from you. The expectations you engender will be reflected in how they respond to your therapeutic efforts.

SUPPLEMENTARY TREATMENT

Should one or both partners have individual therapy in preparation for or as a supplement to marriage counseling? Is medication, sex therapy, or day treatment referral to another agency, such as vocational rehabilitation, indicated? If a husband or wife is acutely depressed, manic, or psychotic, another kind of treatment may be a prerequisite for marital therapy. Sex therapy usually is more effective after some progress has been made in marital therapy on communication and joint problem solving. Minor sexual dysfunctions may often improve with marital therapy alone. There is time in marital therapy to provide exercises, assignments, and feedback on sensate focus, pleasuring, and instructions for alleviating premature ejaculation; however, if the sexual dysfunction is long-standing and primary, specific therapy for the disorder is indicated. Marital therapy and marriage counseling cannot be all things to all patients, and an awareness of their limitations is as necessary as an awareness of their potentialities.

—— • ——

Sybil and Judd are an example of how a variety of services were brought to bear before maximum benefits from marital treatment were realized. Judd was in the navy and the couple had lived in a southern California seaport for only a few weeks before he was sent overseas for 10 months. They both felt that they had made adequate plans for the separation. Base housing had not been available, but a suitable apartment had been found, and Judd had helped Sybil get acquainted with a few other navy wives and with some community resources, including the base commissary, library, post office, and church. Neither had any idea of the extent to which Sybil would feel isolated—even abandoned—in a strange environment. She missed not only her husband but her mother and her sister and her friends, who were all on the East Coast. Her mother had recently married a man Sybil detested, so she felt cut off from her. Her sister was pregnant and the doctor didn't feel she could make the trip west, so Sybil felt forsaken by her, too. This sudden drop in social support resulted in Sybil's withdrawing into her apartment, neglecting to eat, and becoming severely depressed. After losing considerable weight and being unable to sleep for several nights, she shared her unhappiness with a neighbor, who called the local community mental health center. The emergency team from the center made a home visit and arranged for Sybil to spend a few nights at the psychiatric inpatient facility. Sybil had developed such extreme fear of remaining alone that she welcomed the opportunity to get some rest in a protective environment. From there, she was referred to a day treatment center, and Judd was called back on humanitarian leave.

While Sybil was still attending the day treatment center several days a week, Judd returned in a state of confusion. He had no idea what had gone wrong and was unsure of how to react to Sybil's depression. He required several individual sessions in order to feel that the whole clinic wasn't ranged behind her—maybe even blaming him—and to establish his own therapeutic relationship with the social worker. He needed an opportunity to release some of his feelings of anxiety, guilt, and resentment and to learn less angry ways of coping with his wife's depression. When they both expressed readiness, they were accepted in an evening married couples' workshop. The marital therapy was supplemented by a prescribed antidepressant for Sybil, which was gradually discontinued as she began functioning and feeling better. A tentative goal had been for Judd to be released from military service, but with Sybil's newly acquired coping skills and the improvement in their abilities to be supportive of each other, new goals were set that did not include his being released from the navy.

— • —

When Mary and Arthur were being evaluated, it occurred to us that some skills training in effective parenting might be a better intervention to start with than marital therapy because so many of their differences were focused on child management. However, the decision to start with marital therapy was made because of the recommendation of the referral source, the severity of the headache symptom, the motivation of both partners, and the need to improve the fundamental communication between them before they could be expected to cooperate in dealing with any one of their many conflicts constructively.

CHECKLIST FOR GETTING STARTED

1. Have you assessed the motivation of each partner to save the marriage?
2. Have you given each partner ample opportunity to ventilate?
3. Have you established a positive therapeutic relationship with both partners?
4. Have you taken a thorough marital history and relationship inventory?
5. Have you developed a tentative evaluation of the personal assets and deficits of each spouse and of the relationship?
6. Have you acquired enough background information, including their perceptions of their respective parents' marriages, to understand some of their expectations of each other?
7. Have you observed their pattern of interaction?
8. Have you assessed their capacities for empathy?
9. Have you screened for sexual problems?
   a. "How did you first learn about sex?"
   b. "Describe your first sexual experiences."
   c. "What kind of a sexual relationship did your parents have? How did you learn about it?"

d. "What kind of sexual experiences did you have prior to marriage? During previous marriages?"
e. "Do you have any negative attitudes about any parts of your body? Explain."
f. "Do you reach climax? Are there any physical complaints that interfere with sexual enjoyment? Premature ejaculation? Dyspareunia? Does fear of pregnancy interfere with your sexual freedom?"
g. "What sort of contraception are you using, if any? Is it satisfactory to both of you?"
h. "Who initiates sex? How often? Would you prefer a different approach? What would be more satisfactory to you?"

10. Are there clearly understood preliminary treatment goals and objectives?
11. Have you made clear to the couple that from this point on, the focus will be on the present and the future, not on the past?
12. Have you formulated a therapeutic contract that includes fees, time frames, and commitment to attend regularly and complete homework assignments?
13. Have you made arrangements for any necessary prerequisite or supplementary treatment?

STARTING A MARITAL THERAPY GROUP

ADVANCE PLANNING

The recruitment for conducting marital therapy in a group involves more active advertising. If you want couples in addition to the ones selected from your own case load, set the starting date for the workshop far enough in advance to allow you to recruit and screen sufficient couples to have at least three couples and no more than five for the group. Letters should be sent out to your referral sources informing them of the group; announcements should be made to staffs and individual colleagues; notices should be circulated and posted. If you are offering the experience as an educational service rather than "therapy," you might advertise the workshop in local newspapers and on local radio and TV via public service announcements. In recruiting, it is essential that the logistical details be mentioned: when, where, how long, whom to contact, and cost.

FORMAT

Your married couples' group should be comprised of a minimum of three couples to provide sufficient opportunities for modeling, for exposure to different kinds of couples with similar problems, and for the magnified reinforcement that characterizes successful groups. The upper limit should be five couples, since more than that number will not leave enough time for everyone to participate, and there is more of a tendency for subgroups to form. Our experience has shown that 6–10 people offer the optimum environment for full participation and maximum cohesiveness. Since it is likely that at least one couple will have to drop out because of illness, working hours, or baby-sitting difficulties, it is usually safe to recruit six couples, or one more than you can handle. This is particularly true if there is a long time lapse between the end of the initial intake or evaluation and the scheduled starting date. Rather than just leaving the couple on hold, it is wise to see them every week or two for marriage counseling during the waiting interval. Do not be concerned that they will be ahead of the rest of the group. With a head start, they may become good role models for the others and can always benefit from some review and repetition.

You will need to decide whether you want to run an open-ended or closed group. There are advantages and disadvantages to either method. Open-ended groups cut down on waiting lists, may be necessary if your rate of referred couples is low, and provide more flexibility in the number of sessions each couple attends, and the overlap can lead to effective modeling by the more experienced participants. On the other hand, it can be disruptive to group cohesion to have to integrate new couples along the way, and the necessary repetition can become tedious. The new couple may feel strange in entering a group where all the members know each other and might feel much more comfortable in sharing the experience with other new couples where they can all be charter members. The closed group has the advantage of becoming more closely knit, with greater *esprit de corps*. Our experience in working with both types of groups has led to a distinct preference for the closed group.

A limited time span with a definite ending date lends a healthy sense of urgency to achieve goals within the limit set. A 10- to 12-session workshop, with each session lasting two hours, is recommended and is the format used in this book. It can be modified to suit particular groups. For example, groups with several highly verbal members may need more time, as may groups where several are unusually slow in learning some of the exercises, whether because of resistance or because of mental limitations. The last sessions may be scheduled at longer intervals to provide for more time to practice new communication skills. This "fading" procedure is described in Chapter 7 under "Ending Group Marital Therapy."

SCREENING

It is best for one or both of the group leaders to screen all prospective couples, even if they have been previously screened by another worker. The intake and evaluation process should emphasize a positive orientation to the group. You may meet resistance to joining a group, but this may be balanced by those partners, especially husbands, who feel more comfortable in a group situation with other men present. It is up to you to develop favorable therapeutic expectations in each couple for the group or workshop experience. Most couples will be wary and reluctant to enter a group. After eliciting their fears and concerns and allowing them to ventilate them to a reasonable extent, you must deal with their concerns directly and affirmatively. Counter the resistance with the rationale for providing marriage counseling in a group format. If you, as leader, are convinced that the group approach is as good as or better than the individual approach, your prospective clients will also become convinced. If you indicate that they have a choice between group and individual therapy, most couples will take the individual approach; therefore, you must promote your group as the most desirable service available from this therapist. If, after expending all possible efforts at persuasion, a couple still absolutely refuses to join a group, you can then make a referral to another treatment option.

SELECTION

The only contraindications to group participation are a total lack of motivation to save the marriage, inability to listen or to follow simple directions, or unwillingness to comply with the conditions outlined below. The major criterion in organizing a cohesive and mutually facilitative group membership is the "sore thumb" principle. If one spouse as a prospective group member stands out like a sore thumb, that couple should probably be excluded and referred to another group where they will be more compatible or to individual marriage counseling. Characteristics to consider are:

1. *Psychiatric diagnosis.* One schizophrenic with active psychotic symptoms would do poorly in a mixed group but

would benefit from a group where another one or two of the couples contain a psychotic member.

2. *Socioeconomic class.* An unskilled laborer and his wife who have not graduated from high school would do poorly in a group where all of the other couples are college-educated professionals.
3. *Racial–ethnic background.* A black couple may or may not do well in a group otherwise white, depending on the sharing of other socioeconomic variables and values; however, a Mexican couple who speak English haltingly and have a strong identification with Mexican culture will probably do poorly and drop out of an Anglo group.
4. *Age and length of marriage.* A couple in their late 50s who have been married for over 25 years would probably do poorly in a group consisting otherwise of couples in their 20s. However, it is possible and interesting to have a group made up of couples spread out over a wide age spectrum and spanning different developmental periods of married life.

In putting together couples for a prospective marital group, homogeneity and compatibility among the couples on the above background dimensions will enhance cohesiveness, group interaction, and productive work. It is important not to be dogmatic about these dimensions, however. Some married couples have expressed their pleasure in having other couples with some differences from them (e.g., 20 years older) because they could see that the problems they were having could recur repeatedly over the years and would not go away spontaneously. It is a matter of using good judgment in selecting couples who have enough in common to feel relatively comfortable together, at least after the first session or two.

COHESIVENESS

You as leader can facilitate cohesiveness and mutual support by your example and by reinforcing whatever commonalities exist. Remember that as the group leader you are a powerful social reinforcer and that you can prompt verbal expressions of mutual support, interest, and empathy. You can point out similarities in the participants, parallels in their problems, and the complementarity in the resources that they bring to the group. For example, one couple may be strong, effective parents and have good suggestions to make in that area, while another couple may be falling apart as parents but may be very skilled in money management. One participant may contribute humor, another an especially warm kind of feedback. Dimensions of cohesiveness and interpersonal affection grow if the tone is set for them and you selectively reinforce their expression by group members.

VALUES OF GROUP MARITAL THERAPY

Groups provide multiple models for various styles of interrelating and a wide range of behavioral options to emulate or avoid. Exposure is offered to different interaction patterns and to more learning opportunities.

The modeling by other participants is of more value than any modeling by therapists because it is "real" and easier to identify with. Research shows that models with slightly better skills are more effective than models with far superior skills, as the learner finds it easier to identify with the former. As one or two couples start making progress, their reports to the group reinforce their own gains and inspire hope in the other members who are progressing more slowly. Groups offer a safe learning environment as trust develops and couples discover that exploring and experimenting with their own relationship can be interesting and rewarding.

A recalcitrant plumber who wouldn't do his homework in couple therapy did respond when he heard the other men in the group read off their Warm Fuzzies with obvious relish. Another resistant husband was furious with his wife for reporting to the group that he refused to have a vasectomy. After listening to another couple discuss whether they wanted the wife to have a tubal ligation or the husband to have a vasectomy, he changed his attitude completely and was willing to discuss it.

As for the value to you, the therapist, you may have to work as hard or even harder in terms of being alert to what is going on. But the group adds a valuable dimension that is usually more rewarding than other kinds of marriage counseling. There is a momentum, a cohesiveness, and a mutual caring among the members that defy description and make every married couples' workshop a unique and memorable experience. It is less expensive in time and money, but those pluses count less than the satisfaction of seeing so much growth take place among so many in such a short time.

ORIENTATION

In orienting each couple to the workshop, give them a description of what they can expect to happen in the sessions and in the homework. Let them know what will be expected of them. A description of a workshop, "An Introduction to Marital Therapy," is contained in the "Client's Workbook," and they should read it before they come to the first session. Answer any questions they may have and explain the underlying assumptions of the group or workshop. When running married couples' groups, it may be desirable to charge in advance for all sessions, whether attended or not, as an inducement for attendance.

The administration of pretests for assessing the couples' problems is also part of the orientation procedure, and these tests are important for later comparison with the posttests for program evaluation. A recommended questionnaire, the "Marital Adjustment Test," is found in the "Client's Workbook."

CHECKLIST FOR ORIENTATION TO GROUP

1. Have both partners been seen by you or your co-leader and have they verbally acknowledged their interest in becoming part of a married couples' workshop (even if reluctantly)?
2. Have they made a commitment to live together without outside sexual activities for the duration of the workshop?
3. Have they agreed to regular attendance, participation in the sessions, and completion of homework assignments?
4. Have you distributed the handout "An Introduction to Marital Therapy"?
5. Have you collected a contingency deposit?
6. Have you administered pretests?
7. Have you given them the date, time, place, and other pertinent information in writing?

CONGRATULATIONS!
Now you are ready to start your group.

REFERENCES

Stuart, R. B. Behavioral remedies for marital ills: A guide to the use of operant-interpersonal techniques. In A. S. Gurman & D. G. Rice (Eds.), *Couples in conflict: New directions in marital therapy*. New York: Aronson, 1975.

Stuart, R. B., & Stuart, F. M. *Marriage pre-counseling inventory and guide.* Champaign, Ill.: Research, 1973.

Weiss, R. L., Hops, H., & Patterson, G. R. A framework for conceptualizing marital conflict, a technology for altering it, some data for evaluating it. In L. A. Hamerlynck, L. C. Handy, & E. J. Mash (Eds.), *Behavior change: Methodology, concepts and practice.* Champaign, Ill.: Research, 1973.

CHAPTER 3

Planning Recreational and Leisure Time

Many couples coming for marital therapy have problems that stem from poor distribution of their time in recreational and social activities. They may be lonely and isolated as a nuclear family, may have lost their playfulness, may spend too much time together, or may be over-involved with their children. Individuals have different needs for solitude and togetherness. These needs may also change as a couple go through the developmental phases of their lives and their marriage. When the amount of each partner's desired emotional space differs within a relationship, the irritations and frustrations coming from satiation and deprivation can lead to withdrawal.

Starting marital therapy with a review of recreational and leisure time may be surprising to your clients, since they might have so many more serious and important things on their minds. It may even seem a bit frivolous to you, the therapist. But focusing on leisure-time activities can be an effective way to begin from several points of view. In the first place, building social and recreational time together may be all that is needed to repair a torn marriage. Since this is occasionally the case, employing more extensive clinical approaches could be like trying to cure a hangnail by amputating an arm. It is advisable to try the simpler, more parsimonious, and less intrusive treatment interventions first and see if they suffice before raising the level, cost, duration, and effort of further interventions. The least time-consuming method that works for the couple is the best. Beware of the pitfall of overcomplicating or reading more into marital problems than really exists.

Some marriages can be satisfying to both partners despite the continued existence of very obvious conflicts.

In the second place, an early focus on recreation is helpful because it can be significant in your assessment of each partner's behavioral assets. It gives you insights into strengths, such as the couple's capacity for mutual enjoyment, willingness to share, and interest in acquiring new outlets and skills. You can discover how each spouse distributes his or her free time—how much time each spends with her or his own friends, with other married couples, with family, and with children.

A third reason for starting marital therapy in the recreational and social domains is that communication over these areas is less emotionally charged than most other areas. Recreation tends to be more unitive than divisive as a topic of conversation and can be one of the most fruitful avenues to explore with discontented married couples. Because recreation and socializing appear to be simple areas for exploration compared with deep-seated problems rooted in the past, they are often underemphasized or even overlooked entirely. This is unfortunate, as rescheduling recreational and social activities can help to rapidly revitalize a marriage.

—— • ——

The Joneses applied for counseling because they were depressed and were taking it out on each other. They felt they couldn't afford to take any time away from home. They were an elderly couple who took great pride in their home. The work Johnny brought home and Edna's church activities were the only exceptions to the yard work, laundry, marketing, and house repairs which filled their weekends. When asked to develop a mutual recreational activity, their first reaction had been to suggest projects to improve their property. Instead, their marriage counselor gave them an assignment to acquire a hobby they could share that was not related to work around the house. After much discussion, they reluctantly decided on camping. They said it was too expensive and took up too much time, but they chose camping because there was absolutely nothing else they could agree on. Two months later, they reported that their whole lives had changed. They loved camping and were happier than they had been in years. Johnny felt that getting close to nature made the difference in their new relationship, while Edna attributed the change to the opportunity of getting away from the ever-present work at home. They both reported that this new recreation had provided opportunities for serene companionship that they had not experienced before.

—— • ——

Attention to recreational projects helps partners to shift from a problem-focused mental set to a fun focus. Engaging in new, pleasurable activities promotes positive behavioral interactions that compete with conflict-laden interactions. *Recreation* means "creating anew," giving fresh life, diversion, and refreshment of strength and spirits. To incorporate play or shared and mutually enjoyable activities into the lifestyle of a married couple can counteract much of the negative interaction, boredom, and emotional deprivation they are experiencing. Their conversation can become revitalized with joint planning for a trip, a party, tennis, an evening course, preparing for rock-hound expeditions, outfitting a camper, or getting involved in a theater group. These joint projects provide many opportunities to increase the volume of positive interchanges and to set the stage for improving the quality of communication.

Peg and Martin knew the joys of joint recreational pursuits but felt they had lost them forever. They had been ski enthusiasts. They had met on the slopes and skiing had been the focus of all their leisure-time activity. After Peg's car accident, she could no longer ski. She had slipped into a martyr's role, and Martin's enjoyment of skiing was drastically curtailed by his guilt at leaving her home. He felt that it would be tactless to talk about skiing, and she felt totally left out. With help, they worked out a compromise that fell short of the pleasure of their preaccident lifestyle but far surpassed their postaccident slump. Peg now goes to the ski resorts equipped with camera, books, and knitting. Skiing is now a spectator sport for her, but the vicarious pleasure is better than the painful satisfaction of martyrdom. Since Martin is no longer guilt-ridden, he is able to reinforce Peg's interest by admiring her photos and encouraging her to send them to a ski magazine for publication.

A helpful approach to improving recreational patterns is to assist the couple in doing a time budget for distributing their leisure time into four categories of interaction:

1. As individuals
2. As a couple
3. As part of a social group (i.e., with other couples)
4. As a family

It is easy to be misled if you do not adopt this framework. For example, when each partner claims a need for more recreation, you might assume that they are talking about the same thing. However, in reality, he may want to go fishing with the boys while she may want to take the kids to Disneyland, and neither of them enjoys time alone together because they fight all the time. It's dangerous to make assumptions about the use of leisure time. When Jeff said that Diane was so "chicken" about recreation that he had to have most of his fun without her, the therapist assumed that Diane really was timid, or perhaps liked croquet, or only desired leisurely Sunday afternoon drives. However, a few questions revealed that Jeff was giving Diane a bad time for refusing to scuba dive in dangerous waters or to skydive. The third option he gave her was drag racing.

In checking out exactly what each wants, this four-point framework can be used as a guide to see where their recreation requires "shoring up" or redistributing. The distribution of time by each to the four areas shifts and changes throughout the life cycle. Newlyweds usually want more time devoted to themselves as a couple, as do elderly couples who are thrown back on their own resources. The fourth category gets more priority from families as their children are growing up. A couple may seem out of sync when one partner needs more time as an individual because of a certain phase that he/she is going through. Both partners are not going to need or want the same weight to be given to the same categories at the same time. Helping your patients become aware of their individual needs is the first step toward their reaching satisfactory compromises.

RECREATION AS INDIVIDUALS

As an adult, every married person has a need for individual use of leisure time apart from her or his partner. The English novelist Jane Austen wrote, "One half of the world cannot understand the pleasures of the other." There is such a thing as too much "togetherness." Beware of the partner who says, "But I don't want to have my fun away from my spouse. I love him/her so much, I want to be with him/her all of the time." The chances are that the other partner is suffering from feelings of being smothered with too much contact and attention. If so, your identification of needs for emotional space will be seen as helpfully supportive. The "I-don't-want-to-do-anything-without-him/her" syndrome is a kind of self-immolation that is stifling to both spouses.

A person who is overdependent on his/her spouse may need supplementary therapeutic intervention. One such supplement is an assertiveness-training group where independent role alternatives, feedback,

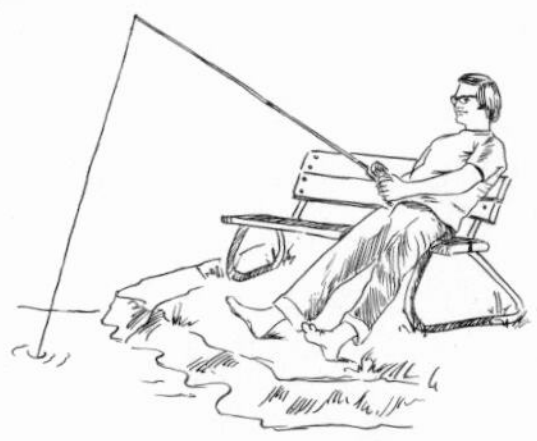

and homework assignments can promote a sense of identity and self-sufficiency that will preclude leechlike dependence on the spouse. There has been a trend in our culture, exemplified by the media, extolling the merits of family cohesion beyond what is realistic or desirable. You may have to be directive in pointing out each partner's need to have space and to be away from each other at intervals. Constructive desire for each other needs time and space to rebuild. As a nursing mother has to separate from her baby in order for her milk supply to replenish itself, so do spouses need a break from each other so their need for each other can be reexperienced. Every couple has a homeostatic balance of interindividual distancing and rhythms of separating and reuniting. When these patterns and rhythms are thrown off balance by overdependency, suspicion, or apathy, a good look at how their time is being used is in order.

— • —

Harriet and Harvey made a contract to have separate annual vacations of at least one week. The couple found that short-term separations resulted in "romantic revivals" that reinforced their individuality. "We each take turns vacating the house for this separate vacation time, which allows the person at home the luxury of the house to her/himself. While I don't think we are unusual in this respect, this tradition feels very comfortable to us and is not accompanied by the resentment I've seen in other couples who attempt separate vacations."

— • —

Fred stopped at a bar every night after work because he had to be alone for a while between office and family. Marilyn, his wife, indicated that she would prefer to keep the children out of his way for 30 minutes after he got home, rather than have him continue to go to the bar. She was willing to take responsibility for ensuring his privacy, even if it meant taking the children out of the house for a walk or play. Fred agreed to try coming directly home, found he liked it, and then spent more of the evening with the family than ever before.

— • —

An American couple is living on a yacht in the West Indies. The wife is counting the months until she can live in a house on dry land again. She explains that she and her husband, the "Skipper," made a long-term recreational contract. As an outstanding golfer, she longed to make the tournament golf circuit, while he longed for the sea. He traveled with her for three years, following her on golf courses all over the country. Now she is his "first mate" for three years. This arrangement is working for them because their contract satisfies their respective recreational needs with support from the other.

— • —

Separate recreation can include being with one's own friends without the spouse. It doesn't mean just solitary recreation. With provision for separate recreation, both partners have choices and time of their own to spend the way they want to. An equitable amount of separateness in recreation can minimize the feeling of not being allowed to lead one's own life. The therapist's task is to guide the partners to find a mutually agreeable and reasonable proportion of leisure time for separate activities. Each couple has to arrive at its own unique compromise. The therapist is only a facilitator. Once reached, reasonable separateness is replenishing and liberating.

Once individual needs for recreation and socializing are recognized, you will have to help the couple communicate these needs to each other in ways that do not leave one or both partners feeling rejected. When there is a clear understanding of needs, an excellent basis for negotiation is established: "If you want to watch football Sunday afternoon, why don't we plan a family picnic for Saturday?" will be more effective than, "Do you have to sit glued to that TV all day Sunday again?" or "Why can't you ever do things with me?" These negotiations and compromises can serve as grist for the contracting mill which will be described in Chapter 6.

RECREATION AS A COUPLE

But too much separate recreation can mean a growing apart. Over and over again, marriage counselors hear, "We don't do anything for fun," "We haven't got the time," or "We can't afford to go out." It is understandable that couples under severe time and financial constraints put a low priority on fun. You may have to point out that a walk doesn't cost any money, nor does a breakfast-in-bed date. And a cup of coffee or tea at a local eatery doesn't take much time or money, either. The planning itself can be a beginning, even if reality pressures

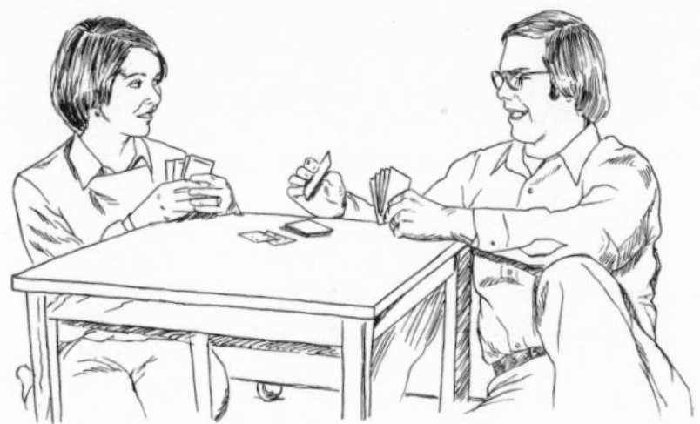

mean a couple of months of "window shopping" before the actual purchase takes place.

Resistance often takes the form of "He doesn't like to do anything I like to do," and "She doesn't like to do anything I like to do." Sometimes tracing back what they did for fun before their marriage yields possible recreational alternatives to TV. You could also make an assignment that each partner list a minimum of 10 recreational pursuits that would have appeal, regardless of time, money, prerequisite skills, or spouse's preference. Encourage them not to be constrained by reality but to fantasize, to take a week to dream up some way-out things they would enjoy doing with each other if there were no holds barred. This assignment can be done on a blackboard, a clipboard, or a bulletin board in your office. The "Guide for Leisure Time Planning" in the "Client's Workbook" may be a source of ideas for the partners. Then you and they can respond with potential compromises that might be worked out. Some examples are:

He	*She*
Fishing	Dancing
Hunting	*Taking a course together*
Photography	Concerts
Tennis	Plays
Skiing	Visiting my family
Watching football	Gardening
Watching wrestling	Shopping
Watching ice hockey	Sierra Club
Playing football	Singing
Wrestling	Ballet

Couldn't they take a course in photography *together*?

When there is very little overlap, it sometimes works wonders to have them alternate in initiating social events for each weekend. He buys the tickets for a game one week, and the next week she plans a photography trip. Another list:

He	*She*
Pitching horseshoes	Sewing
Swimming	Quilting
Rock hunting	Gardening
Mountain climbing	Reading
Camping	Watching TV
Hiking	Embroidering
Fishing	Playing bridge
Collecting butterflies	Flower arranging
Picnicking	*Jewelry making*

A combined compromise of becoming rock hounds and jewelry makers together was the successful outcome for this couple.

Mary and Arthur's list:

Arthur	*Mary*
Bringing company home for dinner spontaneously	*Going for walks*
Family picnics	Listening to records
Cooking together (without my being ordered out of the kitchen)	Yoga
Gardening	Dancing
Camping	Bird-watching
Miniature golf	Going to church
	Stargazing

Combining daytime picnics with walks and evening picnics with stargazing met Arthur's and Mary's needs. Usually you will find ample overlap in these activity lists, which make excellent points of departure for discussion and planning.

One couple with four teenaged children had not spent a night away from their kids in eighteen years. Their homework assignment was to spend a night at an inexpensive motel in a nearby town. They had such a good time that they decided to do it on a monthly basis. This plan had more positive repercussions than they had anticipated. Her depression lifted as a result of having a special event to look forward to each month. They learned that their children could get along without them for brief periods. It also gave them something to plan for, enjoy, and reminisce about afterwards; thus, it became a "core symbol" of their marriage.

Couples must have time by themselves if intimacy is to be maintained. Long periods are not required. Of course, the quality of the time spent is more important than the actual number of hours. But there must be enough private time for relaxed communication on a verbal, affectional, and sexual level for the fulfillment of needs and for the nurturing and replenishing of the relationship.

Here are how some couples have described their efforts to work out a satisfactory plan for sharing time together, and time apart.

> She lets me do the things I enjoy. She doesn't interfere if I want to go someplace or do something on my own. And she expects me to respect her freedom also.

> I have quite a few hobbies that my husband is not involved in. I value the friends and contacts that I make from these activities — weaving, dancing, theater. I like the feeling of being known for myself as an individual, not just part of a couple.

> Because we have some separate interests, we spend some of our leisure time apart. This doesn't seem to be a problem, and we often bring ideas and news back to share with each other.

> Both of us have separate individual interests and hobbies. Once in a while, one of us has to remind the other that he or she is wanting more time together. Sometimes, it's too easy to become absorbed in separate things and neglect family matters.

RECREATION WITH OTHER COUPLES

When encouraging a social life involving other people, you may want to start by looking at whom the couple is associating with, if anyone. Many couples come to counseling feeling lonely, and an astounding number report no friends at all. If this is the case, some basic social-skills training is in order. Participation in a married couples' workshop can be a good transition toward developing friendships. If most of their

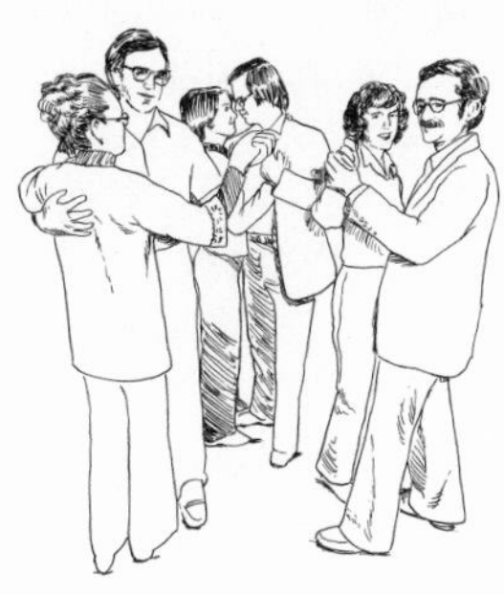

socializing is with her divorced girlfriends, his bachelor boyfriends, or couples who are splitting up, this can have an adverse influence on their marriage, and you may want to encourage them to associate with happily married friends.

Couples usually have an unwritten contract on initiating plans for social activities. It is interesting to learn which partner assumes this responsibility and how they both feel about it. Exploration of this control dimension reveals important diagnostic information and points to training goals.

—— • ——

Mary worked for weeks in an assertiveness training group on being able to respond to social invitations with the statement, "I'll call you back after I talk to Arthur." This ended a long series of conflicts in social engagements, hurt feelings, and arguments about why she accepted invitations without checking with him or the calendar first.

—— • ——

Another wife, Sylvia, had given up on making plans to do things on weekends because, although Tom always went along, he always complained. With help, they clarified that he really wanted her to take the initiative and make most of the decisions about what *to do, but he had definite ideas about* with whom. *He did not like her friends and she didn't like his. After some bitter interchanges, they agreed to reach out together for new friends in new social situations—in a folk dance group, at church, and among a few mutual acquaintances whom they both could accept. This plan worked well for them.*

—— • ——

Jim and Lucille had not been out socially together for two and a half years. He gave as the reason that Lucille would never come home until hours after he suggested it. It was always, "Just one more drink, or one more dance," which then led to seemingly endless conversations. Lucille said that of course she prolonged it as long as she could: "When you get out only every couple of years, you have to make the most of it." A plan was developed for going out at least every two weeks and coming home within fifteen minutes of Jim's suggesting it. Their social life blossomed, adding zest to their marriage. At last report, they were both enjoying going out more than once a week.

—— • ——

A boat can be either a divisive or a solidifying piece of recreational equipment. Lee and Debby had fallen into a pattern where the Windsong *was "his" boat, while their home was "her" house. It took considerable time and work for the boat and house to become "ours." Lee had planned to sail away if the marriage counseling didn't improve their communication, while Debby was steadfastly asserting that her seasickness was a physical illness and not psychosomatic or a hostile act. Among other items, their contract specified a new kind of drug for motion sickness, home repair time to balance boat maintenance time, Debby's right to refuse involvement in boat racing, some joint cockpit entertaining with Debby's assuming more responsibility for the galley, and additional safety measures aboard.*

RECREATION AS A FAMILY

Recreation as a family unit is not easy to work out because of the variety of tastes and needs at different age levels; however, it is of major importance to marital harmony and family solidarity. Many families spend too much of their hard-earned leisure time in routine visiting of grandparents, where habits have become ingrained, precedents for celebrating holidays are unbreakable, and boredom or bickering are the order of the day. Variety and creativity can break these patterns in ways that are to everyone's advantage. Even the grandparents, who everyone assumes are only too happy with things as they are, will often welcome changes in routines.

There can be problems with the extended family that seriously interfere with family recreation. For some couples, interference from parents and/or in-laws becomes a divisive issue in which one partner or the other really suffers from feelings of split loyalties. Others live in a kind of uneasy peace with parents and in-laws. And some get on quite well with "the folks" and genuinely enjoy their company. It is

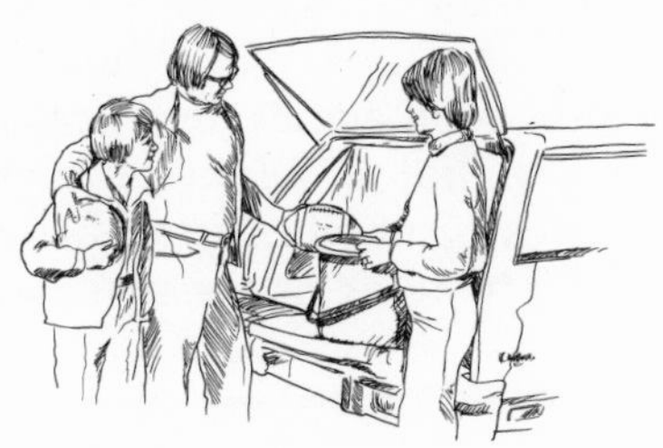

your job as therapist to help the couple bring about some resolution of conflicts with extended family relations. It may happen that a grandmother's baby-sitting has to be sacrificed in order to preserve the couple's independence and privacy. An interfering mother-in-law who feels that she has a right to be a part of all of the couple's social life may have to be dealt with assertively. It has been said that when a man marries, he must divorce his mother. Jim's mother gladly accepted a referral to a senior citizen recreation program. On the other hand, with another couple, Darryl had to change the locks on their doors to prevent his mother-in-law from walking in unannounced at any time. If the couple can learn to communicate with each other about how and when they want to include the extended family in their recreational plans, then they can present a united front to the grandparents, aunts, or cousins. They can gain control of their own time and make their own choices.

A couple can use marriage counseling as an opportunity to take stock of their involvement as a family in recreation. Perhaps an assignment to have other family members participate in the activity-listing assignment described above will be fruitful. Or, perhaps, if the children are getting into their teens, they need more opportunities to be with their peers, and an honest reappraisal of where everyone is "at" will be the beginning of new recreational pursuits. Actually, this was not a problem area with Mary, Arthur, and their daughter, Lisa. They all enjoyed family outings.

Family night, as recommended by churches, can be a time for mutually enjoyed leisure time. It means that all family members make a commitment to devote one evening a week to discussion, reading aloud, music, games, or joint hobbies. It's an inexpensive program in time and money, and if there is sufficient motivation, it can be rewarding for all involved. Teenagers who would much rather be with their peers may need extra incentives to participate. Once a family has successfully instituted a recreational plan, all members will feel challenged to plan activities that are satisfying to everyone. Such activities can include pulling taffy or making homemade ice cream, if nostalgia and sweets have appeal. Other familywide possibilities include growing a garden, making improvements on the house or the garage or the yard (and then celebrating the achievement), barbecuing, bicycling, badminton, Ping-Pong, swimming, jigsaw puzzles, word games (anagrams, Scrabble, Perquacky), number games (dominos, Monoploy), sorting family pictures for hanging or albums, jewelry making, or various forms of charades.

Families may want to make changes in the way they split up for entertainment, too. Sister may want to go to the ball game with Dad, and Sonny might like to go plant shopping with Mom. A breaking out of role stereotypes to sample a broader repertoire of recreational options can be a positive stimulus to individual growth and family interaction.

Your work in this area needs to be highly individualized for each couple and may well include some family therapy sessions with the children and even with other relatives. The important thing is to be sure to include in marital therapy an examination of the couple's social and recreational use of leisure time.

In the group or workshop format, inputs about recreation are made richer and more stimulating by the variety of people present. Couples often follow examples set by other participants when activities are described with enthusiasm. One couple took up racquet ball, another jogging, and two couples even joined a swim club as a result of discussion during the sessions. Participants in groups seem to be more open to accepting the importance of carving out satisfying recreational patterns for themselves and their families. They are full of suggestions for potential compromises and for trying new things. Reports of recreational adventures usually provide some comic relief, and the time devoted to the discussion of recreation is usually well spent. It is conducive to the cohesiveness of the group and to concrete, positive, mutual planning by the respective couples.

CHAPTER 4

Communicating: Awareness of Reciprocity

INTRODUCTION

Good communication is essential for healthy couples. Communicating feelings and transmitting information are the keys to a satisfying relationship and the cement of the marital union.

Partners communicate with each other in a variety of ways. They talk and they touch, smile and cry, come together and withdraw. When communication between partners is direct and honest, when there is a free flow of feelings and ideas, each partner serves as a speaker and a listener with the other. Each partner gives and asks for emotions, information, suggestions, opinions, agreements, and disagreements. How effectively a couple communicate feeling and facts in a reciprocal way determines the amount of satisfaction or distress in a marriage.

Exchanging personal messages in a marriage requires skills that have frequently never been learned or, if learned, are all too easily neglected. Our experience has been that most couples cite problems in communication as their principal cause of marital discord and as the major motive for participating in therapy. Marriage counselors and therapists have the task of teaching couples constructive and mutually helpful ways of communicating facts, desires, opinions, feelings, and unmet needs.

Teaching communication skills must focus on everyday, mundane interaction as well as on rarer moments of intimacy. As we pointed out in the previous chapter, couples who enjoy doing things together and who have compatible time budgets for distributing their social and leisure activities have an important source of union. Similarities in values, preferences, and personal habits can also contribute to the strength of a union. But the mechanism for energizing and maintaining a union comes from effective patterns of communication between husband and wife.

From our experiences as marital therapists, we feel that the teaching of communication skills—listening as well as expressing—is by far the most important feature of successful treatment and counseling of couples. Spending two chapters on "communication" reflects our priorities and felt importance. Our attention is on both the rational and the emotional dimensions of communication. The French philosopher Blaise Pascal wrote, "Le Coeur a ses raisons, que la raison ne connaît pas"—the heart has reasons that reason does not understand. Emphasizing this same quality in our time, Albert Ellis has termed his particular approach to therapy "rational–emotive." Reason and emotion are complementary and essential in human interaction.

There are two primary components to communication in marriage: the verbal and the nonverbal, what is said, and how it is said. Communication can become aversive if, for example, a partner uses an accusative verbal style of expressing anger, "Why do you always act so helpless and stupid?" Even more often, however, communication gets fouled up because the verbal message gets lost in the nonverbal medium of expression. Nonverbal communication by means of tone of voice, facial expression, gestures, and body posture may be more important than the actual words used.

One couple told us how important nonverbal communication was for them: "We use nonverbal signals during sex and in ordinary affection. Maybe he gives me a pat on the head or I may hold his hand. If that kind of thing is missing, tension builds up and we lose contact with one another. Then things between us can get bad. When the affectionate nonverbals start again, everything quickly becomes better." We will direct your attention to both dimensions of communication and provide exercises for couples to increase awareness and improve the quality of verbal and nonverbal interchanges.

Effective communication enhances marital happiness. It has been said that marriages are *not* made in heaven—neither is marital happiness. A good relationship is the result of each spouse's having needs met through reciprocity. Affecting reciprocity, or its converse, coercion, are many factors, some of which may be easy to identify while others escape detection. Sometimes reciprocal communication and a fully satisfying mutual relationship may come about without any conscious attempt to reach this goal. Spontaneity is beautiful when it happens! But often planning and purposeful action are necessary to facilitate open and positive communication, particularly by the time a distressed couple comes to you for therapy or counseling.

The following fairy tale by Dr. Claude M. Steiner illustrates this point very well. Dr. Steiner is the author of *Scripts People Live* (1974), a transactional analysis approach, in which effective communication is viewed as one of the most important elements in psychotherapy. We recommend that you tell this fairy tale to your clients or patients early in therapy or at a time when they are worried about "spoiling" their partner by engaging in too much positive communication.

A FAIRY TALE: WARM FUZZIES

Once upon a time, a long time ago, there lived two very happy people called Tim and Maggie with two children called John and Lucy. To understand how happy they were, you have to understand how things were in those days. You see, in those days everyone was given at birth a small, soft, Fuzzy Bag. Anytime a person reached into this bag, he was able to pull out a Warm Fuzzy. Warm Fuzzies were very much in demand because whenever somebody was given a Warm Fuzzy it made him feel warm and fuzzy all over. People who didn't get Warm Fuzzies regularly were in danger of developing a sickness in their back which caused them to shrivel up and die.

In those days it was very easy to get Warm Fuzzies. Anytime that somebody felt like it, he might walk up to you and say, "I'd like to have a Warm Fuzzy." You would then reach into your bag and pull out a Fuzzy the size of a little girl's hand. As soon as the Fuzzy saw the light of day it would smile and blossom into a large, shaggy, Warm Fuzzy. You then would lay it on the person's shoulder or head or lap and it would snuggle up and melt right against their skin and make them feel good all over. People were always asking each other for Warm Fuzzies, and since they were always given freely, getting enough of them was never a problem. There were always plenty to go around, and as a consequence, everyone was happy and felt warm and fuzzy most of the time.

One day, a bad witch became angry because everyone was so happy and no one was buying potions and salves. The witch was very clever and devised a very wicked plan. One beautiful morning the witch crept up to Tim while Maggie was playing with their daughter and whispered in his ear, "See here, Tim, look at all the Fuzzies that Maggie is giving to Lucy. You know, if she keeps it up, eventually she is going to run out and then there won't be any left for you!"

Tim was astonished. He turned to the witch and said, "Do you mean to tell me that there isn't a Warm Fuzzy in our bag every time we reach into it?"

And the witch said, "No, absolutely not, and once you run out, that's it. You don't have any more." With this the witch flew away on a broom, laughing and cackling all the way.

Tim took this to heart and began to notice every time Maggie gave a Warm Fuzzy to somebody else. Eventually, he got very worried and upset because he liked Maggie's Warm Fuzzies very much and did not want to give them up. He certainly did not think it was right for Maggie to be spending all her Warm Fuzzies on the children and on other people. He began to complain every time he saw Maggie giving a Warm Fuzzy to somebody else, and because Maggie liked him very much, she stopped giving Warm Fuzzies to other people as often, and reserved them for him.

The children watched this and soon began to get the idea that it was wrong to give up Warm Fuzzies any time you were asked or felt like it. They too became very careful. They would watch their parents closely and whenever they felt that one of their parents was giving too many Fuzzies to others, they also began to object. They began to feel worried whenever they gave too many Warm Fuzzies. Even though they found a Warm Fuzzy every time they reached into their bag, they reached in less and less and became more and more stingy. Soon people began to notice the lack of Warm Fuzzies, and they began to feel less warm and less fuzzy. They began to shrivel up and, occasionally, people would die from lack of Warm Fuzzies. More and more people went to the witch to buy potions and salves even though they didn't seem to work.

Well, the situation was getting very serious indeed. The bad witch who had been watching all of this didn't want the people to die (since dead people couldn't buy his salves and potions), so a new plan was devised. Everyone was given a bag that was very similar to the Fuzzy Bag except that this one was cold while the Fuzzy Bag was warm. Inside of the witch's bag were Cold Pricklies. These Cold Pricklies did not make people feel warm and fuzzy, but made them feel cold and prickly instead. But, they did prevent peoples' backs from shriveling up. So, from then on, every time somebody said, "I want a Warm Fuzzy," people who were worried about depleting their supply would say, "I can't give you a Warm Fuzzy, but would you like a Cold Prickly?" Sometimes, two people would walk up to each other, thinking they could get a Warm Fuzzy, but one or the other of them would change his mind and they would wind up giving each other Cold Pricklies. So, the end result was that while very few people were dying, a lot of people were still unhappy and feeling very cold and prickly.

The situation got very complicated because, since the coming of the witch, there were less and less Warm Fuzzies around; so Warm Fuzzies, which used to be thought of as free as air, became extremely valuable. This caused people to do all sorts of things in order to obtain them. Before the witch had appeared, people used to gather in groups of three or four or five, never caring too much who was giving Warm Fuzzies to whom. After the coming of the witch, people began to pair off and to reserve all their Warm Fuzzies for each other exclusively. People who forgot themselves and gave a Warm Fuzzy to someone else would immediately feel guilty about it because they knew that their partner would probably resent the loss of a Warm Fuzzy. People who could not find a generous partner had to buy their Warm Fuzzies and had to work long hours to earn the money.

Some people somehow became "popular" and got a lot of Warm Fuzzies without having to return them. These people would then sell these Warm Fuzzies to people who were "unpopular" and needed them to survive.

Another thing which happened was that some people would take Cold Pricklies—which were limitless and freely available—coat them white and fluffy and pass them on as Warm Fuzzies. These counterfeit Warm Fuzzies were really Plastic Fuzzies, and they caused additional difficulties. For instance, two people would get together and freely exchange Plastic Fuzzies, which presumably should have made them feel good, but they came away feeling bad instead. Since they thought they had been exchanging Warm Fuzzies, people grew very confused about this, never realizing that their cold prickly feelings were really the result of the fact they had been given a lot of Plastic Fuzzies.

So the situation was very, very dismal and it all started because of the coming of the witch who made people believe that some day, when least expected, they might reach into their Warm Fuzzy Bag and find no more.

Not long ago, a young woman with big hips born under the sign of Aquarius came to this unhappy land. She seemed not to have heard about the bad witch and was not worried about running out of Warm Fuzzies. She gave them out freely, even when not asked. They called her the Hip Woman and disapproved of her because she was giving the children the idea that they should not worry about running out of Warm Fuzzies. The children liked her very much because they felt good around her and they began to give out Warm Fuzzies whenever they felt like it.

The grownups became concerned and decided to pass a law to protect the children from depleting their supplies of Warm Fuzzies. The law made it a criminal offense to give out Warm Fuzzies in a reckless manner, without a license. Many children, however, seemed not to care; and in spite of the law continued to give each other Warm Fuzzies whenever they felt like it and always when asked. Because there were many, many children, almost as many as grownups, it began to look as if maybe they would have their way.

As of now it is hard to say what will happen. Will the grownup forces of law and order stop the recklessness of the children? Are the grownups going to join with the Hip Woman and the children in taking a chance that there will always be as many Warm Fuzzies as needed? Will they remember the days their children are trying to bring back when Warm Fuzzies were abundant because people gave them away freely?

RECIPROCITY IN COMMUNICATION

Marital communication involves three steps: (1) awareness and recognition of messages coming in from your partner; (2) cognitively processing those messages and developing ideas for possible responses; (3) sending back your own messages with their verbal and nonverbal components. This chapter will help you work with couples to enhance their reception skills, their sensitivity to the positive messages, or events (PLEASES) that occur in marriages. The next chapter will cover listening skills and strategies for responding to and sending messages. But first, let's review how marital communication can be subverted or effectively used by partners to achieve their emotional and material needs.

Personal, social, and material needs can be met or approximated in various ways, some of which are effective and desirable and some of which, like coercion, are harmful and destructive.

COERCION

The spouse who uses coercion gets fulfillment of needs by making life unpleasant enough for the partner to have the latter give in, comply, or accede to requests and demands. Unpleasantness is escalated until compliance is won. Each spouse gives in to the other to avoid or escape from unpleasant interactions, threats, annoyances, or arguments. This is a typical case of negative reinforcement; giving in is reinforced because it stops unpleasant experiences. In this situation, both spouses are likely to obtain fulfillment of some of their needs, possibly even satisfaction of several needs to a significant degree—but the satisfaction comes as a hollow victory and at a great cost to the relationship. With intimidation, a spiral occurs, with each spouse taking turns as temporary victor and victim.

—— • ——

Our prototypical couple, Mary and Arthur Peabody, displayed coercion in the following exchange:

Mary: *Arthur, we have to buy a new sweater for Lisa.*
Arthur: *What? Again? Only last week you bought her clothes, and she still has that green sweater.*
Mary: *Last week, I bought her a dress, and that green sweater is much too heavy for now—that's winter clothing.*
Arthur: *There's always something else to buy! Why can't you shop more carefully? We simply can't afford it.*
Mary: *Why do you always have to complain? I've worked all day and I'm getting a headache.*
Arthur: (Shouting) *We cannot afford it, and that's that!*
Mary: *O.K., simmer down. I won't buy the sweater. But you're not going to win the next argument we have.*

—— • ——

In this coercive interaction, Arthur "wins" because no money is spent. However, Mary will have her turn at being the coercing partner next time. In playing the coercion game, both gain some satisfaction from the forced compliance of the other, but one can hardly speak of this as producing a mutually satisfying fulfillment of needs.

NEGATIVE EMOTIONAL RESPONSES

Paradoxically, giving and receiving negative emotional responses may sometimes be a major force that keeps the couple together. By *negative emotional responses* we mean those words, expressions, and actions that are experienced as unpleasant, for example, insulting remarks, crying, an angry tone of voice, hostile silence, sarcastic comments, put-downs, and ridicule.

Negative emotional responses may at first glance appear to be punishment that might be expected to turn a partner off and kill a relationship. However, getting a rise out of your spouse by engaging in provocative or annoying behavior is better than no response at all and can actually be a powerful source for maintaining a relationship. When there is a paucity of pleasant interactions, as when spouses take each other for granted, one partner will settle for any kind of emotional response from the other, even if it is negatively toned and unpleasant. These negative emotional responses tend to reinforce or strengthen the unpleasant behavior that evokes them, and thus another spiral is set into motion. One partner's anger or outburst provokes a similar response from the other, which, in turn, keeps the angry tirade going.

Let's see how Arthur and Mary use negative emotional responses with each other to sustain their communication.

—— • ——

Arthur: *We are way over the budget again!*
Mary: (No response—silence.)
Arthur: *Can't you find a less expensive supermarket? The food bill is atrocious.*
Mary: *Stop eating for a while. That will save you money and me time.*
Arthur: *Don't be asinine. I'm trying hard to save, and I don't get any support from you.*
Mary: *If I'm that stupid, you go and buy the groceries. If you do that, as well as taking care of Lisa, we'll soon be in good financial shape.*
Arthur: *You could at least find the specials in the store!*
Mary: (Getting angry, pretending to speak to herself, but making sure Arthur hears) *Now, let's see, for dinner, we will have bread. And I guess we can afford water . . .*
Arthur: (Leaves the room, slamming the door.)

RECIPROCITY OR PLEASES

While it is true that coercion and negative emotional responses can maintain a relationship and even enable spouses to obtain some of their needs, it is pleasant interaction that creates strength and satisfaction in the marriage bond. When spouses do and say things that please the other, they experience the relationship as rewarding and will be eager to enjoy each other's company more often. Pleasant words and actions, which we usually call PLEASES or Warm Fuzzies in this manual, include such varied items as pleasant smiles, attentive listening, expressions of appreciation, considerate requests, and thoughtful surprises. Flowers and candlelight dinners are well established as international PLEASES, but even very small tokens, such as a warm "thank you" or an unexpected hug, can be enjoyable and effective PLEASES. When both spouses frequently give PLEASES to each other's personal, social, emotional, and tangible needs, a positive spiral is started in which the PLEASES of one spouse reinforce the PLEASES of the other.

— • —

Let's look in on Arthur and Mary again and see how they use reciprocity in their communications. Arthur has just arrived at home, a bit late from work.

Arthur: *Hi, Honey, sorry I'm late, but it was a busy day at the office.*

Mary: *That's quite all right. I don't have dinner ready yet. Lisa had some trouble with her math homework and I tried to help her.*

Arthur: *OK, you take care of dinner and I'll see if I still know that math.*

Mary: *Thanks! I know you must be tired, but Lisa will be happy if you help her.*

Arthur: *Lisa, let me help you and then after dinner, we'll both help Mother with the dishes.*

Mary: *That would give me a chance to iron your shirts so you'll have a clean one for tomorrow.*

— • —

After this conversation, dinner is still not ready and Arthur is still tired, but chances are that family harmony has increased. Mary has help with the dishes, Arthur gets a clean shirt, and Lisa can finish her homework. Even more importantly, all are aware of each other's needs and use PLEASES *to satisfy these needs.*

— • —

There are a number of ways to structure the marital therapy so that the couple can learn to use PLEASES more frequently in building reciprocity in their communication and relationship. In the rest of this chapter, we will describe such procedures as reciprocity awareness, "Catch Your Spouse Doing Something Nice," love days, fantasy fulfillment, and core symbols. However, you should feel free to create and develop exercises and instigations of your own that will have the same effect, namely, the acceleration of pleasing exchanges in the marriage.

In proceeding with this section on reciprocity, remember that we are:

1. Taking responsibility for structuring the therapeutic environment to promote active learning
2. Starting with positive communications before getting involved with the more difficult area of expressing negative feelings

RECIPROCITY AWARENESS EXERCISE

Couples who request marital therapy frequently demonstrate an astonishing lack of awareness of the pleasant things one spouse does for the other. Pleasing behavior, PLEASES, or Warm Fuzzies are taken for granted or have become so routine that all life seems to have gone out of them. All too often, both partners are so wrapped up in their respective problems and dissatisfactions that the positive elements are pushed into the background. Therefore, you, as the therapist, will want to start therapy by teaching and training those communication skills that PLEASE each spouse. The "Client's Workbook" that accompanies this book has specific instructions for completing the homework assignments on PLEASES, including sample lists of PLEASES. Your first step is to acquaint and familiarize your couple with the concept of a PLEASE.

This reciprocity awareness exercise, used by many marital therapists to get the ball rolling with positive interactions, was described in a publication by Azrin, Naster, and Jones (1973). You ask each spouse to list 10 PLEASES that he/she is giving to the other and 10 PLEASES being received from the other. PLEASES are defined simply as any word, expression, favor, routine, or action of one that pleases the other. This can be done in the session on notepaper or a blackboard. You can also give this exercise as a homework assignment during the first session or even at the end of the evaluation period in anticipation of the first session.

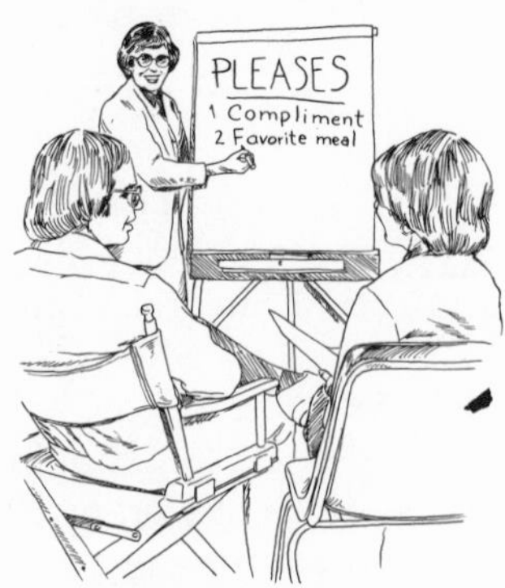

When the lists are completed, have each spouse read aloud the 10 PLEASES currently being *given to* the partner and the 10 PLEASES currently being *received from* the partner. One purpose of this exercise is to teach the couple how to *specify* their interactions in concrete and observable terms. Thus, as they read their lists, be sure to help them translate any vague or general PLEASES (e.g., "My wife loves me") into descriptive, discrete, behavioral language (e.g., "My wife gives me a hug and kiss when I come home from work"). It is all right for both spouses to list the same activity—for example, "taking a peaceful walk in the country"—if it was shared by both. Help the couple reach agreement on the accuracy, nature, and frequency of the stated PLEASES. This process will begin to build shared meanings and perceptions and reduce distortions and unfounded expectations. One partner might surprise the other by divulging interactions and activities that the other had no idea were rewarding or pleasing. Take such opportunities to point out how they can increase their marital satisfaction by simply reporting more often what they like about each other. Of course, reinforce their PLEASES by commenting on them, asking them to elaborate them in greater detail, and expressing your own pleasure in hearing about them.

It is important to start the reciprocity awareness exercise and assignment from the very first treatment session. As soon as the evaluation and catharsis stages are over, you should teach the spouses to direct their attention to the nice and pleasant things they do and say to each other. When, under the direction of the therapist, the marriage partners take a fresh, positive look at their interactions, significant progress can be made in a relatively short time.

You might want your clients to review the examples of PLEASES from the exhaustive list provided in the "Client's Workbook." This will give them a clearer idea of what constitutes a PLEASE and will illustrate the importance of being specific. A very effective technique is also to give examples of PLEASES from your own life and marriage, so that the spouses learn a wide variety of possibilities and understand that nothing is silly or unimportant. The spouses are prompted to identify PLEASES that are relevant for them and are already occurring in the marriage. You may have to restrain a spouse from making negative comments such as, "If only he would do that!" or "That she never does!"

After the couple have identified PLEASES that are important to them, you may emphasize again that these are not requests or demands but rather statements of pleasant events that are actually occurring. You may ask each spouse to mention two or three of the PLEASES being given and received that are particularly important. (Limiting the number of PLEASES mentioned helps maintain a positive atmosphere.) In encouraging verbal reflection on PLEASES, you should avoid awkward silences, get the partners to talk directly to each other, and cut off any remark that may color the PLEASE with a negative hue or a put-down.

HUSBAND: *(To the therapist.)* She is a good cook.
THERAPIST: Don't tell me—tell your wife!
HUSBAND: I like the way you cook dinner.
WIFE: Thank you.

HUSBAND: You cleaned the kitchen yesterday, and I like that because usually it is a big mess and . . .
THERAPIST: *(Interrupting.)* Stop! Mention the pleasing item, but don't turn it sour. Say that again and stop after "I like that."
HUSBAND: You did the kitchen yesterday and I like that.
WIFE: Thank you.

WIFE: He says he likes it when I balance the checkbook, but he always complains that I spend too much money.
THERAPIST: Do that once more. Now, look at your husband and start with "I like it when . . . " Also, leave out the negative remark at the end.
WIFE: *(To her husband.)* I like it when you tell me that . . . uh . . . that you are pleased when the checkbook balances.
HUSBAND: It takes a load off my mind.

The main purpose of this exercise is to make each spouse aware of what is liked by the other and to promote actions that are pleasing to each other.

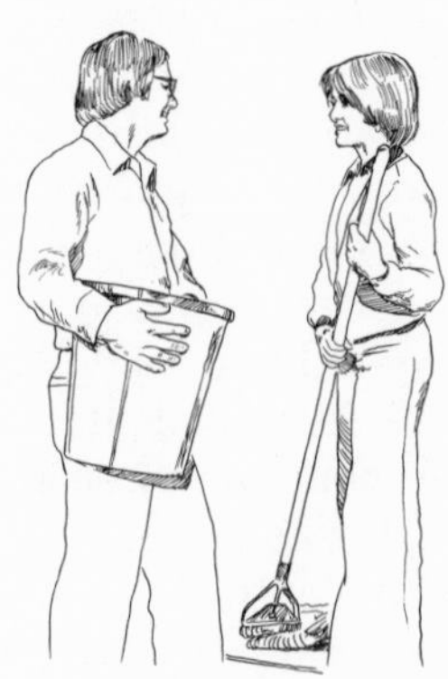

CATCH YOUR SPOUSE DOING SOMETHING NICE

This exercise and homework assignment, developed by Dr. A. Jack Turner, should become a regular part of each therapy session. You ask the spouses to note and record daily at least one PLEASE received that day from the other. The PLEASES are written down and then shown to each other at the end of the day. Exchanging records lets each spouse find out what he/she did that was appreciated by the other and serves as a reinforcer for the PLEASE. Because of the show-and-tell method of exchanging PLEASES, this exercise might be better called, "Catch Your Spouse Doing Something Nice and Let Him/Her Know About It." It is important that these recordings be made each day and not all at the end of the week, because daily recording increases mutual attentiveness to each other's pleasing behavior. It is very common for partners to want to drop this task after a few sessions. They may claim that they know how it works, that it becomes repetitious, that many good things happened, but that they do not recall exactly what. You, as the therapist, should insist that your clients faithfully complete the assignment "Catch Your Spouse Doing Something Nice" each day. Overlearning facilitates spontaneity, and behaviors that are easy to comprehend are often hard to do. Besides, lots of wrong practice in the past may necessitate thorough training in the present. It would be wise for you to have the couple thoroughly and correctly practice this exercise in your office before trying it at home. If the assignment is done in the wrong manner at home, away from the watchful eye of the therapist, the marriage may erode further. When the couple returns for their next appointment, you may want to vary their reporting of the "Catch Your Spouse" assignment to maintain daily interest and involvement in the exercise. For example, you might ask them to report:

- The most important PLEASE.
- The PLEASE which was a complete surprise.
- The times he/she said something nice.
- The times she/he did something nice.
- The PLEASE which was very personal.

In the "Client's Workbook" are a number of forms entitled "Catch Your Spouse Doing Something Nice" (see Figure 2, p. 76). These forms should be used for the daily recording of PLEASES.

The exercise "Catch Your Spouse Doing Something Nice" (see Figure 2) provides you with opportunities to inject more positive reactions into different arenas of the marital relationship and helps the spouses to increase their daily happiness. We have found in our marital therapy

CATCH YOUR SPOUSE DOING SOMETHING NICE

NAME__________ NAME OF SPOUSE__________

DAY	DATE	PLEASING BEHAVIOR
MON.		
TUES.		
WED.		
THURS.		
FRI.		
SAT.		
SUN.		

Figure 2

that the recording of PLEASES can affect almost any situation. For example, here are some reports made by Mary and Arthur on their catching each other doing or saying something nice!

INCOME

Arthur: *Mary, your part-time job helps the money squeeze we're in now. I really appreciate it that you asked for some extra hours this month.*

Mary: *Thank you.*

Mary: *You know, Arthur, I feel very secure with you because you are such a good provider.*

Arthur: *That's nice of you to say so.*

BUDGETING

Arthur: *You did a great job managing our money this week, Mary! With all the bills for gas and electricity, I never thought we'd make it.*

Mary: *Thanks, Arthur, I really tried.*

Mary: *I liked it, Arthur, that you suggested buying that new rocking chair yourself. I knew that you had been saving, but I didn't think we could afford it.*

Arthur: *You deserve it, Honey.*

—— • ——

CHILDREN

Arthur: *I was so proud of the way the teachers talked about Lisa at school. Your helping her with math has paid off.*

Mary: *Thanks—and I'm pleased that you came with me to the school.*

—— • ——

Mary: *You helped me a lot, Arthur, when you took Lisa to that party. I was so busy, and Lisa was afraid she was going to be late.*

Arthur: *Anytime.*

—— • ——

SEX

Mary: *That was a real surprise when you made reservations at that expensive resort for our anniversary! I felt so wanted.*

Arthur: *I'm glad you liked it so much.*

—— • ——

Arthur: *Mary, you make me feel so good, letting me be myself when we're making love. I especially like it when you rub my chest.*

Mary: (Responds with a kiss.)

—— • ——

AFFECTION

Mary: *When you hug me, Arthur, I feel so close to you. You really let me know you care.*

Arthur: *I do care.*

—— • ——

Arthur: *When you kiss me when I wake up, Mary, I always have to smile because I know you love me.*

Mary: (Smiles)

—— • ——

HOUSE CHORES

Mary: *Thanks for repairing that leaking faucet, Arthur. It's been irritating me for several days, but I didn't want to ask you because I knew you were busy.*

Arthur: *No problem, Mary.*

———•———

Arthur: *Heavens, Mary, how can you get those big windows so clean? There's not a streak on them!*

Mary: *Thanks! You really notice the difference, huh?*

———•———

MEALS

Mary: *Breakfast in bed last Sunday! Arthur, you make me feel like a queen when you do that!*

Arthur: (Smiles)

———•———

Arthur: *Mary, your pies are out of this world. I especially liked the cherry pie you made yesterday!*

Mary: *You can expect another one Sunday!*

———•———

As indicated in the examples, the spouses should acknowledge the pleasing action or expression clearly and directly when it occurs as well as when they share and exchange diaries with each other at the end of the day. A simple "thank you" will usually suffice, but you may also find it useful to have the clients practice alternative and comfortable ways of acknowledging PLEASES in your office. We suggest that you, as the therapist, ask the clients about their reactions to receiving PLEASES. Part of the pleasure in giving PLEASES comes from being acknowledged for extending them to others. Acknowledgments and feedback will further strengthen the couple's reciprocity. For example:

———•———

HUSBAND: I liked it when you had dinner ready early today.

WIFE: Thank you.

THERAPIST: (To wife.) *How did it feel when your husband gave you that* PLEASE?

Or:

WIFE: It relieved me when you took the trash out this morning.

HUSBAND: Sure, I worried it was piling up.

THERAPIST: *(To husband.)* How do you like the compliment your wife gave you?

Both spouses are to keep their own individual list of PLEASES on the form "Catch Your Spouse Doing Something Nice." These daily recordings are regular assignments and typically continue for as long as the therapy sessions last. It is strongly recommended that you actually collect the lists of PLEASES during each session, since this reflects your serious interest in the homework and will motivate the clients to do the assignments. At the beginning of each session, you, as the therapist, can request one spouse to read the list of what the other did or said that was pleasing. Then ask the other spouse, who gave the PLEASE, whether this pleasing event was acknowledged. Since most people like to hear good things about themselves, the reading of PLEASES will create a positive atmosphere for the remainder of the session.

GROUP MARITAL THERAPY

The exercise "Catch Your Spouse Doing Something Nice" is excellent for groups. The members will stimulate each other to find new pleasing behaviors, learn new expressions that PLEASE, create variations within existing pleasing patterns, and thank their spouses for the PLEASES. Less creative members can get suggestions from others. If a given PLEASE did not work out very well, others can usually come up with suggestions for improvements. If one or both partners come to a group meeting without having done their homework on keeping a record of PLEASES, then you can turn to the others who did and allow them to serve as constructive models for the "delinquent" partners. Reasons or excuses for noncompletion of homework are not reviewed or discussed so as not to reinforce resistance and noncompliance. Perhaps the greatest advantage of a group setting is practicing communication in front of others and seeing others do it, too. The sharing of PLEASES and the observation of other couples' interactions facilitate generalization of the behavior learned in the therapist's office to the everyday setting.

After about four sessions of charting PLEASES for "Catch Your Spouse Doing Something Nice," the couple may be given a homework assignment to double or triple the number of PLEASES normally given one day during the coming week. These days are called *love days* and are not to be announced to one's partner. The spouses are to report back in the following session on what happened and whether the love day was actually noticed by the recipient. These PLEASES need not be spectacular events, but small services and considerations that each spouse knows will please the other. Some examples are a few extra hugs and kisses, cooking a special meal, offering to watch the children for half an hour, saying "I love you" more often, washing the dishes, or servicing the car. To instigate this exercise, you can assign a love day to each spouse each week. The "Client's Workbook" has assignment forms for this purpose. After a few weeks, the partners can pick their own love day spontaneously.

The "Catch Your Spouse Doing Something Nice" and the love days homework assignments are important parts of therapy for a couple, and you need to facilitate their completing these assignments. It is crucial that you review the homework assignments with the couple to demonstrate their importance to the couple and to provide the opportunity to reinforce the couple's efforts. During homework review, encourage the spouses to describe the PLEASES received from each other and how it made them feel when PLEASES were given or received. It has been our experience that most couples report warm, good feelings regarding the giving and receiving of PLEASES during the week. Occasionally, in the first weeks, a couple will say that this process felt "forced" or "mechanical." If this should happen, emphasize that it usually takes time for the pleasurable feelings to begin to accompany the *actions* of giving and getting PLEASES. Encourage them to continue with the assurance that the mechanical aspects of going through the motions will eventually be replaced by spontaneous, natural, good feelings. During homework review, ask each spouse how his/her partner verbally and nonverbally *acknowledged* receiving a PLEASE. Ask the couple if they are beginning to feel that they are getting more positives from each other. Emphasize that each can also ask for PLEASES at will, for example, "I would really like a hug right now."

When a couple has been successfully recording and acknowledging PLEASES for several weeks, you may give them the option of not continuing with the formal charting of PLEASES. The purpose of the charts is to instigate and accelerate the exchange of PLEASES and may become superfluous if the couple is able to maintain a high rate of pleasing exchanges, because reciprocity has become firmly implanted and naturally reinforcing. Some couples may wish to continue using these charts voluntarily as a helpful prompt or reminder to give and acknowledge PLEASES. Do not discourage the continued use of the charts if one or both spouses wish to continue using them.

What do you do when a couple does not complete the homework on PLEASES or does it only sporadically? Explain in a matter-of-fact way that they will get out of the therapy only what they put in and that the homework assignments are a very important component of the therapy. Try not to preach or criticize, as this may inadvertently reinforce their resistance. You might arrange to call them on the phone between sessions to remind them of the assignment. This helps to bridge the gap from session to session and underlines the importance of the assignment.

When one spouse is completing the "Catch Your Spouse Doing Something Nice" sheets and the other is not, you should encourage that person to express her or his hurt and anger in direct ways, as will be described in Chapter 5. Also, reassure the complaining spouse that each person moves at his or her own rate and that patience is necessary. Ignore "martyred" feelings and encourage and reinforce the faithful spouse to continue completing the homework. Refocus the couple on positive changes that have occurred in their relationship.

PERFECT MARRIAGE AND FANTASY FULFILLMENT PROCEDURE

Another exercise that can generate greater awareness of reciprocity is the perfect marriage and fantasy fulfillment procedure developed by Azrin and his colleagues (1973). This may be carried out over three sessions, or if more time is devoted to it, it may be completed in a single session. Here's how the procedure works.

Ask the couple to write down eight problem areas for married couples: sex, communication, child rearing, money, leisure and social activities, household responsibilities, job, and independence–dependence. You may also put the list on a blackboard or a poster to help focus their attention. Without consulting the other, each spouse is asked to write down fantasized desires that would make their marriage "perfect" in each of the problem areas. Instruct the couple to be as selfish as possible in stating their fantasies. Their desires need not be reasonable or realistic since they will be used by the therapist as starting points to formulate new interaction patterns.

Using the fantasied interactions from the perfect marriage lists, each spouse is asked to pick and say aloud one new desire that would significantly improve the marriage. Next comes the fantasy fulfillment stage. As the therapist, you help guide the couple to negotiate and develop a compromise so that their respective fantasies can be realized, at least in some small measure. This requires active shaping by the therapist to transform and approximate each spouse's fantasy into a reality that can produce positive feelings. Here are some examples:

One husband, who wanted total independence and fantasied owning an island and being completely autonomous, agreed to spending the next weekend camping out on an island near their home. A woman said she would have a sexually perfect marriage if her husband would run nude with her across a field of flowers, plunge into a mountain lake, and then make love under the sun. With some prompting from the therapist, she and her husband agreed to find a secluded spot in a local park and use it for lovemaking. Another wife, who fantasied a round-the-world cruise, agreed, as an approximation, to spend a day touring the old passenger liner, the *Queen Mary*, moored as a public attraction in the city of Long Beach, California.

To assist a couple in compromising on the actualization of a stated desire or fantasy, you may translate the fantasy into a continuum of possible activities in terms of frequency, duration, or situation. Seeing desires and hopes on a continuum rather than in an all-or-none character can facilitate compromise and agreement. For example, if a husband stated his fantasy for more independence and time to work on his hobbies, the therapist might translate this vague goal into the explicit dimensions of the performance of the activity: How often do you want to work on your hobbies or be separate from your wife? For what length of time? Where do you want to enjoy this independence? Perhaps after these reality-based questions are answered, the husband and wife would agree to his spending 30 minutes, three times weekly, in the basement or the garage working on hobbies. After an agreement has been made on how to approximate fulfillment on one or two of the fantasies for a perfect marriage, the spouses should be given an assignment to try out the exchange of these fantasies. At the next session, ask them to describe how fulfilling the assignment was. If the couple reports success and satisfaction, the therapist should reinforce them by reflecting back the positive report and by eliciting further elaboration on the event and its associated feelings.

If one or both partners fail to complete the assignment, do not criticize; instead, constructively work toward remedying the lapse. You can always give a person praise for effort or for even thinking about the assignment. This positive feedback from you will encourage future effort. You can also help them fulfill their fantasies by:

1. Having them choose another fantasy from a less sensitive problem area.
2. Scaling down the agreement to a more modest approximation of the fantasy; for example, instead of a wife's agreeing to initiate sex once a week, she might agree to initiating a hug or kiss. Use the dimensions of frequency, duration, time, and place in scaling down a fantasy to more realistic and attainable levels.
3. Teaching the couple to be more *specific,* concrete, and operational in their descriptions of what they want and are willing to give to or do for each other.

The perfect marriage and fantasy fulfillment procedure is one way for the partners to learn that they can have the kind of marriage they desire if they "think small" and settle for realistic approximations of their ideal.

CORE SYMBOLS

Core symbols offer another basis on which to develop positive interactions and to emphasize the reciprocity that exists in a relationship. A core symbol, as delineated by Richard B. Stuart, is any event,

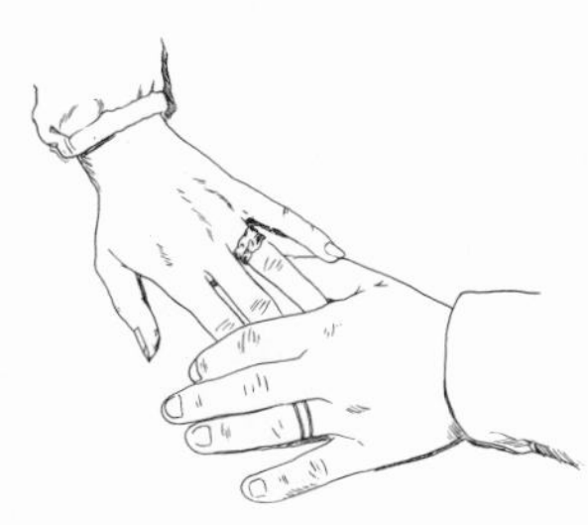

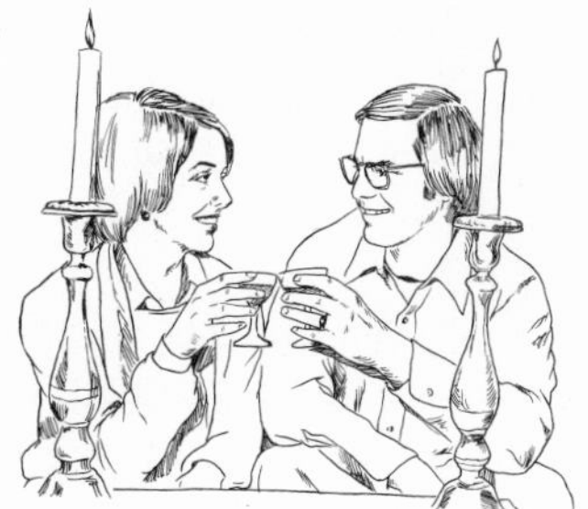

place, ritual, or object that carries special meaning for the relationship to both marital partners. Core symbols are usually experienced regularly—every anniversary, New Year's Eve, monthly, or annually—and bring back warm, positive memories of mutual love, romance, shared joy, and affection. A special song, the honeymoon, the place where they met, pictures, eating by candlelight, and wedding rings are examples of core symbols of a marriage. When core symbols are violated—as when one spouse takes off the wedding ring in anger or refuses to participate in one of their rituals—the whole relationship is jeopardized.

One couple described how their marriage survived a disastrous honeymoon, which made the honeymoon a core symbol to them. They had eloped at the age of 16 and had driven to a motel on four bald tires with no spare and not enough money to buy a decent meal. They had three flat tires and engine trouble and ran out of gas. The whole trip had been one misadventure after another. Out of the discussion with the therapist, an assignment evolved to reinvigorate their honeymoon as a core symbol. They were to make a return visit to the same motel, in style this time, and focus on how much they had gone through together and how much better off they were. So the place of their honeymoon began to represent, along with the humor of the situation, more and more positive associations as an affirmation of how much they had grown together. Even aversive memories can be "reframed" so that they feel uniting rather than divisive. Their jalopy became their beloved clunker with a personality of its own. A tiny replica of an antique car was a new gift to themselves because of what it symbolized to them.

Souvenir collectors can usually come up with quite a few core symbols, but any couple can come up with something. An adult show-and-tell of core symbols can be therapeutic and a lot of fun; an old shoe that was tied to the bumper of the car at the wedding, the audio tape of their wedding ceremony, anniversary pictures, articles of clothing that were worn on special occasions. If the search means ransacking the attic or garage, so much the better if it leads to recalling and valuing articles representing the potential they had hoped for in their marriage.

———— • ————

A special time can have meaning, too. Arthur and Mary had fallen into the habit of designating Friday evenings as a time they would spend together, just the two of them. When they first started to go together, Arthur used to pick up Mary at the school where she taught, and they would go to a beer garden and drink beer and sing old Ger-

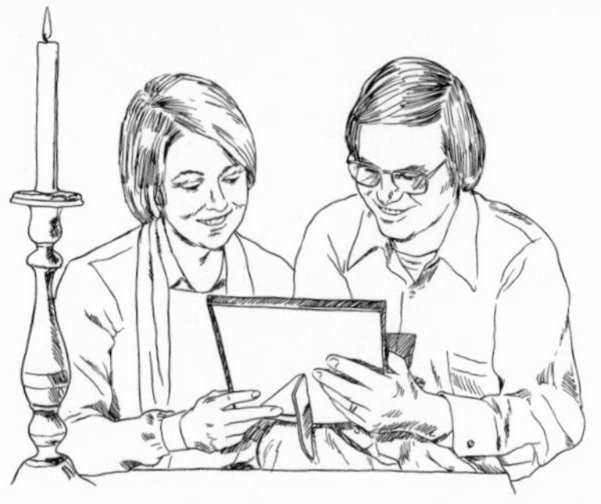

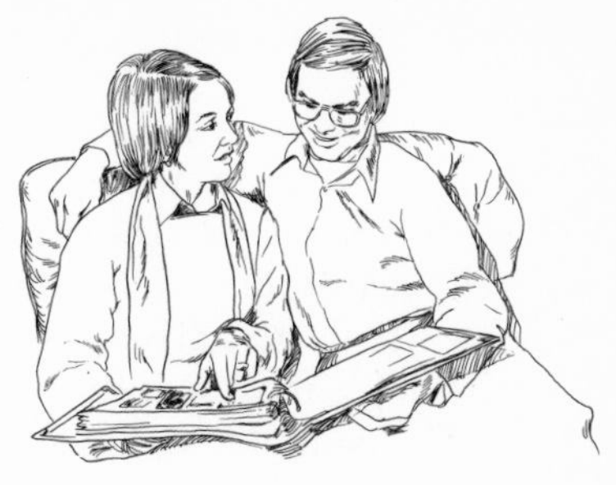

man songs. Their relationship was richly supported by the core symbols that came out of that shared experience when they were falling in love. Some German songs, a decorative beer stein, German beer gardens, and Fridays all meant something special to them.

They had spent their honeymoon at a beach town with a long pier out into the ocean. There had been some seals on some rocks near the end of the pier that caught their interest. Arthur had carefully explained to Mary that the seals couldn't jump from the rocks or climb down, so they were waiting for high tide to get back into the water. Right at that moment, the seals all leaped or dove into the water. When Arthur gets patronizing in his explanations, Mary reminds him of this incident, and since the experience is so embedded in positive associations, he can accept her chiding. Their honeymoon generalized to the point where a walk on any pier and the sight of any seal are core symbols because they evoke such warm, mutually shared memories.

—— • ——

In addition to objects, places, and times, rituals belong to the core symbol category. Larry and Joan made ice cream together, experimenting with a wide range of exotic flavors. Their "ice cream breaks" were intimate, shared times set aside for closeness. Dan and Francie devised an elaborate monthly Sunday candlelight supper with wine and music in front of an open fire to fulfill the assignment of developing a core symbol. Patio suppers with the same accoutrements had already been planned for warm weather. Gustatory rituals work well: breakfast in bed on Sunday mornings. Liqueurs in bed at night, cooking together, and picnics can all come to mean special events to be anticipated and enjoyed with relish. These events forge strong marital links and are the stuff of which family traditions are made.

Hymn singing, meditation, massage, tennis, or an activity that brings the partners close to nature as well as close to each other are effective core symbols. To belong to a large organization as a pair, whether as a Sunday school teaching team or a bridge partnership, can also serve the same purpose. Joint memberships as dance partners, parents, or a couple in mixed doubles on the tennis court have value that transcends the basic recreational uses described in the last chapter.

To recapitulate once more, a core symbol can be a thing, a place, a time, a ritual, an activity, or a way that a couple define themselves. Core symbols may be introduced at any time in the course of treatment. They are invaluable as a way of helping couples get in touch with their positive feelings in relation to the marriage that may have been buried deep under layer upon layer of hostility and discouragement.

GROUP THERAPY

As a means of strengthening the exchange of PLEASES, the couples in the group are asked to share out loud their core symbols. If a couple cannot identify a core symbol, they are encouraged to develop one with each other. Reminiscing in the group often leads to remembering more core symbols or to identifying special events, places, or mutually shared items or songs as core symbols.

When the couples in the group were invited to share their core symbols, Peggy and Philip said they didn't have any. Peggy said, "That's why we're here. We don't have anything to hold us together or to make our marriage special." Philip said, "Well, we do have that special song." Peggy blushed and replied, "We're not going to tell them *that!*" Naturally, the curiosity of the other group members was aroused. After some good-natured coaxing, Peggy said sheepishly that their special song was "I Can't Get No Satisfaction." Dissolved in the laughter of the group's reaction was the pessimism of Peggy and Philip toward their marriage.

SUMMARY

For the therapist conducting marital therapy and reestablishing a couple's communication, the task is to help each partner become more sensitive to the wishes, desires, and needs in the relationship. Awareness of reciprocity is the very foundation of communication between the spouses; communication of reciprocity encompasses words as well as actions, verbal as well as nonverbal expressions, and both the rational and the affective domains. When needs remain unmet, dissatisfaction is unavoidable. When pleasing each other is again a major objective, the marriage becomes alive and love is reborn.

The fairy tale demonstrates that Warm Fuzzies cannot be replaced by Cold Pricklies, and even Plastic Fuzzies do not do the job. Giving Warm Fuzzies or PLEASES in a love relationship entails a risk. It is worth taking such risks if mutual trust and awareness of reciprocity exist in the marriage.

Awareness of reciprocity necessitates that one look beyond oneself. When one learns to catch one's spouse doing something nice, Warm Fuzzies are increasingly exchanged, and a positive relationship is strengthened. Orienting partners toward what the other does that PLEASES, rather than toward what causes friction, is an essential part of therapy. We recommend that awareness of PLEASES be an integral part of each therapy session. Once complaints are transformed into compliments, grudges can become loving requests.

Two special techniques that promote the awareness of reciprocity are the perfect marriage and fantasy fulfillment procedure and the search for core symbols. The spouses learn to look for positive things within their own relationship and to discover the elements that make their union a special and precious one.

The next chapter focuses on communication as the art of listening and as the art of expressing oneself effectively. Once awareness of reciprocity has been established, a favorable atmosphere is created for training to begin on a wide range of communication skills.

REFERENCE

Azrin, N., Naster, B. J. & Jones, R. Reciprocity counseling: A rapid learning-based procedure for marital counseling. Behavior Research and Therapy, 1973, *II*, 365–382.

Steiner, C. M. *Scripts people live.* New York: Grove, 1974, pp. 107–110.

CHAPTER 5

Communicating: The Arts of Listening and Effectively Expressing Feelings

For effective communication, both what we say and how we say it are important. Becoming aware of the PLEASES that are wanted by a spouse is a tremendous step forward in the communication process, but knowing what to say without the ability *to transmit* the message can transform intended PLEASES into bombshells. In this chapter we explore the skills of listening and expressing that determine personal effectiveness and marital satisfaction.

As you observe your married clients express to each other their likes and dislikes, their desires and needs, you will often discover that they don't convey their feelings directly or clearly. Ineffective communication blocks the sharing of beautiful moments and opportunities for greater intimacy, and worse, leads to conflict, to feelings of rejection and withdrawal. Table I has examples of common roadblocks to effective communication.

Emotional expression is not taught in schools. We learn it incidentally from role models, such as parents, siblings, and friends, and from the corrective interpersonal feedback our fledgling communication attempts receive. The interpersonal skills that our married couples demonstrate are acquired more by accident than by design. Part of our responsibility as marital therapists is to design a therapeutic program that can promote the learning of good verbal and nonverbal communication. With a systematic and structured training program, couples can learn to improve their ability to communicate directly, congruently, empathically, and supportively. Training focuses on the messages and how they are sent—on the content and style of communication, rather than on the *why*. Asking "Why did you (or I) do or say that?" frequently leads to intellectualization, rationalization, frustration, or friction. Learning to express feelings effectively requires practice in therapy sessions and also at home. Repeated practice is the soul of learning.

TABLE I. Roadblocks to Effective Communication: Destructive Messages

1. Ordering. "You get in here and clean up this mess right now!"
2. Threatening. "If you don't get in here this minute, there'll be no more TV tonight."
3. Moralizing. "It's your responsibility to clean up after yourself."
4. Providing solutions. "Why don't you start cleaning up during the next commercial break?"
5. Lecturing. "You'll have to learn to clean up after yourself if you ever want to make a good wife."
6. Criticizing. "You never finish anything you start."
7. Pseudoapproval. "I can see you're too tired to clean up this mess tonight."
8. Reassuring. "You'll feel much better once you take care of this mess."
9. Ridiculing. "You're nothing but a slob."
10. Analyzing. "You're just doing this to make me mad."
11. Interrogating. "Can you give me one good reason why you can't clean up now?"
12. Withdrawing. "I'm too tired to argue anymore. I'm going to bed."

THE COMMUNICATION PROCESS

Communication involves *receiving*, *processing*, and *transmitting* information and requires the existence of three elements: the sender, the receiver, and the message. Dyadic communication can be ineffective when any one of these three elements is lacking. Attention to all three elements may help to explode a common misconception among marital partners: each partner tends to assume that her or his sending of a message is okay but that the reception is awry. The communication process can be conceptualized as including:

1. Receiving the message: listening accurately and determining the other's feelings and intent
2. Processing the message: putting the message into context, thinking of response options, and weighing the respective consequences of each option
3. Sending back a message: timing your response and using verbal and nonverbal skills

Most clients go through a series of stages when they learn to improve their communication skills:

- *Confusion*. There is a realization that something is not working right, but the person is at loss as to what it can be. Random attempts are made toward improvement, but usually only greater confusion and frustration result.
- *Awareness*. Explanation and demonstration by the therapist brings about a recognition that there are various styles and degrees of communication. The spouses understand that the receiver, the message, and the circumstance all place certain demands on the sender.
- *Awkwardness*. The couple attempt new modes of communication but realize that they fall short of the model observed during the awareness stage. The spouses initially may perceive themselves as phony, which often makes them want to drop the exercise or defer practicing the skill at home. During this stage, lots of coaching and training in the therapist's office, followed by carefully structured homework assignments and feedback, can overcome the awkward, artificial feelings.
- *Proficiency*. Gradually, the clients acquire the various skills and enjoy the mastery of the newly learned techniques. However, they still feel a definite self-consciousness when the skills are used, and they have to force themselves to implement the techniques. This is perhaps the stage where you, as the therapist, have to be most forceful; practice and consistent home-

work assignments are required to prevent the spouses from stopping halfway.

- *Integration*. The communication skills are no longer associated with the therapist's office but have become part of each spouse's mode of operation. They feel like "me" and not like something imposed from the outside.

ACCURACY AND CONGRUENCE IN COMMUNICATION

Good communication occurs when the actual effects on the listener are the same as the speaker's intended effects. It is not sufficient for the speaker to have the right intention; rather, the listener has to receive the message as it was meant by the speaker. As the therapist, you may want to start by modeling an exercise, which ensures that congruent communication will occur. For example, you and one client could do the following role play:

THERAPIST: You're home early today.
CLIENT: You said that I am home early today.
THERAPIST: Is dinner ready?
CLIENT: You asked if dinner was ready.

Stress that the client is to repeat both the *content* and the emotional tone of the message. The *feelings* aspect of a message is important and cannot be presumed by the content alone. For instance, the message "Did you remember to send flowers for my mother's birthday?" may be taken as a simple direct question of whether a request was remembered or, alternatively, as an implied doubting of the spouse's concern for the mother-in-law. It all depends on *how* the words are spoken and the speaker's facial expression. Thus, the sending of the message is important in communicating meaning.

You may also want to clarify how even simple statements or questions can be easily distorted or misinterpreted by the receiver of the message. Instruct each spouse to say such things as:

- "Dinner is really good today."
- "The work at the office went smoothly."
- "Did you finish that letter to *X*?"
- "Have you seen today's paper?"

After the client speaks, react in a clearly correct or incorrect manner; for example:

CLIENT: Dinner is really good today.
THERAPIST: You mean that it is not good on other days?

or

Thank you for that compliment!

or

I'm glad you liked it!

It is advisable to avoid sensitive topics and to exaggerate clearly when modeling negative ways of sending, receiving, and processing communications. Usually, the spouses will get the idea pretty rapidly. Once the discriminations between congruent and incongruent communications are demonstrated, you can have the couple role-play with each other while you provide prompts or act as a coach in other ways:

HUSBAND: Have you seen today's paper?
WIFE: *(After prompting by therapist.)*

1. Yes, it's in the kitchen.
2. Yes, I'll get it for you.
3. No, I really haven't.
4. No, I thought you had it a moment ago.
5. Why are you always losing track of things?

It is important that the couple realize that both content and feeling have to be accurately received. Therefore, you may want to instruct one spouse to portray a given feeling tone—surprise, happiness, wonder—and then have the other spouse interpret the message. It is wise to wait before using examples of negative emotions until the couple master positive feelings first. Modeling and feedback help to facilitate active participation by the clients. As an example, you can have the spouses take turns delivering and then describing messages and their feeling tone:

HUSBAND: Did you finish that letter to *X*?
(in a surprised tone)
(in a happy tone)
(in a neutral, questioning tone)

The wife is then instructed to state the feeling she perceived.

After some time, start introducing longer segments of conversation. Here, the technique of *doubling* may prove to be useful; that is, you sit close to one of the spouses and, taking his or her role momentarily, demonstrate various ways to send, receive, and process messages.

Here is an example of a therapist doubling for both the husband and the wife:

HUSBAND: The work at the office went smoothly.
WIFE: Did you have a good day, huh?
HUSBAND: Yes, I finally finished that account that kept me busy for three days.

WIFE: *(Silence.)*
THERAPIST: *(Prompting the wife.)* Ask if this is an especially busy time for your husband.

or

THERAPIST: *(Doubling for wife.)* I get the feeling that we only talk about your work. I'd like you to ask me about how my day went.

To promote a greater sensitivity to the other person's needs and, thus, better "receiving" skills, you may ask the spouses to exchange positions. Role reversal provides an opportunity to experience the other person's situation and feelings. To create as lifelike a situation as possible, the spouses should actually exchange seats.

WIFE: I went to that new shop today.
HUSBAND: How did you like it?
WIFE: It looks very attractive, but the arrangement is not clear.
HUSBAND: I'm not sure what you mean.
WIFE: *(Explains what she means.)*

After a few minutes of interchange, ask the wife to take the place of her husband and vice versa. The whole conversation is then repeated. You will want to start out with a neutral topic, but after some training, pleasant items can be discussed. Prompting and feedback will often prove necessary, but the spouses usually enjoy the experience and will contribute more and more elements of their own. Bringing their own response styles and real-life topics into the role plays, the spouses ease the generalization from practice in the therapist's office to their actual daily lives.

Throughout these exercises, which should be spread over several therapy sessions, the clients are assigned homework in order to practice at home the skills learned in therapy. These homework assignments are essential, since it will take time and effort before the proper communication skills are acquired and strengthened. Initial success in your office will bolster the spouses' confidence, but it may also prematurely and erroneously lead them to think they have reached their goals. Additional training via homework assignments, followed by reports on their home-based experiences during the next session, provides you with the opportunity to give support, suggest alternatives, and correct mistakes.

In the discussion of the content and the feeling of a message, it has been stressed that correct communication means that the message is received as it is intended. Miller, Nunnally, and Wackman (1975) pointed out that the frequent complaint that one's partner does not communicate is a fallacy. There *is* communication, but the message may be unclear or may appear contradictory, hostile, or evasive. One example from their book depicts a young couple studying for exams:

> Pam looks up from her book and says, "Jack, let's take a break now. Maybe we can go over to Cicero's and get a pizza. Want to?"
>
> Jack grunts but continues to read. Pam moves over next to him and scratches the back of his neck. "Are you ready to take a break now?" Jack doesn't reply and continues to read.
>
> . . . for Pam, the problem is how to unscramble the silent coded message. Does Jack mean, "Go away and leave me alone?" Or does he mean, "Wait until I finish reading this page?" Or perhaps he means, "Coax me a little more" or maybe even, "You know I don't like pizza—I'm going to hang tight until you suggest hamburgers."

Problems arise from trying to uncode silent and unclear communications. It is often necessary to teach a couple how to convey and receive information accurately. Miller *et al.* suggested that accurate awareness of sending and receiving messages consists of five dimensions. They arranged these five elements into an "Awareness Wheel" (see Figure 3).

If we know what we do, what we want, what we feel, what we think, and what we sense, we can communicate messages better and are more likely to obtain our desired response. Perceptions can become more accurate in marital therapy and distorted perceptions can be corrected.

You may want to focus on each dimension separately to promote awareness:

DOING *(Describing one's behavior.)*
"I didn't suggest going out for dinner last night because I had a headache. What about going today?"

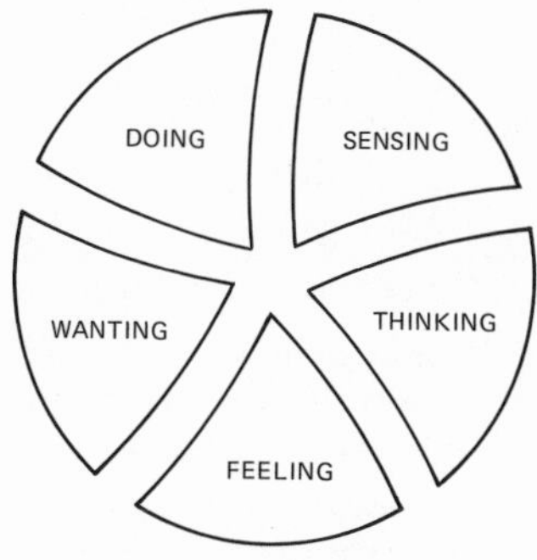

Figure 3

WANTING (*Describing one's intentions.*)
"I would like to go out for dinner tonight."
"So would I, but we really can't afford it."

FEELING (*Describing one's emotions.*)
"I'm in a good mood and would like to go out for dinner. I'd like you to come, too."
"I'd sure love to! Am I ready for a steak!"

THINKING (*Describing one's interpretations.*)
"You seemed disappointed when we didn't go out for dinner last night."
"You got the point—I sure was!"

SENSING (*Describing what one sees, hears, and touches.*)
"Don't you want to go out for dinner? You seem hesitant and have a frown on your face."
"I want to go, but I don't know what to wear."

When spouses describe their behaviors, intentions, emotions, interpretations, and senses, they should not assume that their partner will understand and know what is being said. Awareness should be practiced through reflecting back and checking out the messages that are received. Correct perception and processing of messages requires training in the therapist's office and a good dose of coaching and feedback, plus homework assignments.

GROUP THERAPY

The same teaching and therapy techniques may be used in group therapy. You should start out by modeling the desired behavior. Slow progress is advised, especially at the beginning, since you should direct yourself to the couple with the least skills. After modeling by you and your co-therapist, a couple who appear more capable in the communication skill in question should be asked to demonstrate the behavior. You will find that positive support and careful coaching will help this couple demonstrate their skills to the group. The various couples are then invited to practice the skill together while you and your co-therapist move from couple to couple, providing support, coaching, and prompting where needed. If interference and roadblocks are encountered, you may want to step in and assume the role of the spouse who is experiencing the problem. However, you should keep in mind that at this stage of practice, all couples need the therapist's attention. After sufficient time for practice has elapsed, ask each couple to offer suggestions and alternative approaches. The therapist should be careful not to get drawn into theoretical discussions or lengthy personal reminiscences but to keep the verbal interchange goal-directed and, if possible, interspersed with modeling by various couples.

Homework should be assigned to the couples in the group as described in the later sections of this chapter. At the beginning of the next session, ask all couples to report on their progress. No time or only limited time should be given to those couples who did not complete or at least try to do the assignments. Compliance with your assignments should be rewarded; therefore, direct your attention and support to those who completed their homework. In a friendly and matter-of-fact manner, encourage the "delinquent" couples to listen to others report on their homework and to make a better effort the next week. All clients are invited to contribute in terms of suggestions, support, and feedback, as these increase cohesion and learning opportunities.

NONVERBAL ELEMENTS OF COMMUNICATION

Because *how* we express our feelings often conveys more emotional tone and meaning than *what* we say, working on the nonverbal elements of expression is a very important part of marital therapy. Couples should directly experience how it feels to give and receive given messages in various ways. The following brief exercises are most effective if the marriage partners interact with each other. You should model the behavior when the couple is not responding constructively.

VOCAL VOLUME AND TONE

Select a very neutral message, such as: "It is nice weather today" or "There are flowers in the park" or "Green is a beautiful color." It is important that the message be a simple statement, not a question requesting a response or an order expecting a reaction. The statement should be brief so that it can be easily remembered and, most importantly, the message should not have any personal overtones.

After a given message is selected, ask the couple(s) whether there are any personal connotations in this statement or whether it is really a neutral sentence. After agreement has been reached that indeed some truly neutral statement has been selected, instruct the spouses to face each other and say the selected sentence in various ways, as you indicate. Each time one spouse says the statement a given way, the other spouse is asked to indicate the nonverbal message received. The roles are then reversed, with Spouse A making the statement and Spouse B translating the nonverbal message into words.

You can give the instructions regarding vocal volume orally so that both partners know what is expected, or you may prefer to write the instructions on small pieces of paper so that there is an element of surprise. The instructions may include:

1. Use a neutral tone of voice.
2. Make the statement a question.
3. Make it a demand.
4. Pronounce it as a reproach.
5. Say it in a loud voice.
6. Louder still!
7. Shout it.
8. Whisper the message.
9. Make it sound as if you are shy.
10. Imitate the tone of being afraid.
11. Try to express an invitation.
12. Sound very casual.
13. Now try being indifferent.
14. Express care, concern.

More variations may be added; as a matter of fact, the more nuances of vocal tone and volume experienced, both as speaker and as listener, the better. Some clients may have problems expressing the finer shades of meaning. You can model these, but you should be very patient with progress. It is better to drop a certain task than to give the couple a sense of failure. Be sure to have the clients realize that they are at all times dealing with a neutral statement and that all meaning is sent and received via vocal volume and intonation. Ask what tone of voice they like best and have them indicate why, for example, "That makes me feel important" or "Now I feel he/she cares about me." Stop any comment referring to previous negative experiences, such as "I never knew she could sound that nice" or "If only he would do that at home, but there he only hollers!"

EYE CONTACT OR LOOKING

Another neutral statement is selected. The marriage partners are now requested to say this new statement to each other, maintaining as much as possible a neutral tone of voice but varying eye contact according to the instructions listed below. Again, feedback is provided by the other spouse:

1. Look the other straight in the eye.
2. Look away completely.
3. First, make eye contact and then break it.
4. First, no eye contact, then make contact.
5. Look hard, demanding.
6. Soften the intensity of your eyes.
7. Look at your toes.
8. Look slightly above your partner's eye level.
9. Turn your head away, but maintain eye contact.
10. Make many brief eye contacts.

In addition to the vocal and eye-contact aspects of nonverbal communication, the following elements of body language deserve attention:

- Facial expression
- Gestures and use of hands
- Body posture
- Pacing and fluency of speech

Exercises for the last four elements of nonverbal communication can be constructed and practiced in ways similar to those used for the first two. After a basic performance level has been reached, have the clients practice combinations of two or more elements:

- Looking away and whispering
- Leaning toward the other, glowering with a menacing facial expression, and shouting and shaking a fist
- Extending arms, palms up, smiling, raising eyebrows, using full tone of voice while making a polite but urgent request

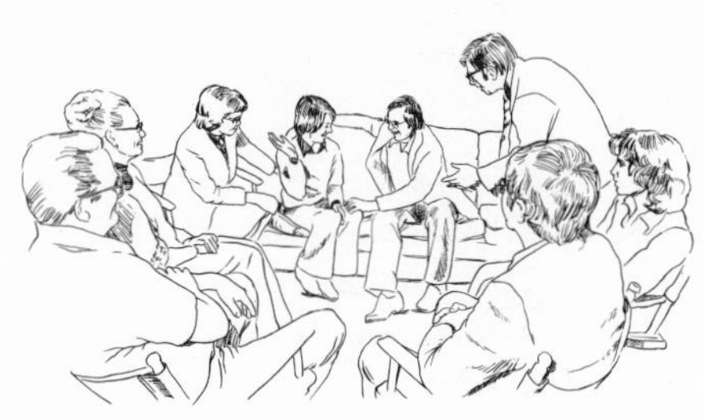

MARITAL GROUP THERAPY

The teaching of nonverbal communication skills is often easier in a group setting than with a single couple because the group members can learn from each other. Support, feedback, and suggestions from all group members should be encouraged.

Suggested group exercises include:

1. One couple demonstrates a given behavior; for example, variations in vocal volume can be illustrated by one spouse saying, "May I have some coffee, please?" All others in the group report how they perceive the speaker and the listener. Then, another couple models and all group members again provide feedback.
2. If one particular couple experiences a given problem, say a lack of facing each other directly, other couples can tell how they approach this situation and thus offer alternatives to the couple experiencing the problem. Modeling by the clients for each other seems especially relevant here.
3. In teaching the impact of facial expression and eye contact, couples may engage in an exercise by forming a circle with one person in the middle. This person then slowly turns around and experiences the reactions of the others in the circle while the others first look at him/her with eye contact and smiles and then later with eyes averted and frowns.
4. Let one couple act out a certain situation without using words, for example, coming home at night and greeting each other or asking for a cup of coffee. Then, ask all group members how they perceived the situation, especially regarding the feeling tone.
5. Let one couple give a "script" of a given situation, for example, asking for a dance or saying "no" to a request. Have another couple rehearse and model the accompanying behavior in front of the group. Then, feedback from all members of the group provides for reinforcement of successful efforts.

When working with several couples in a group, it is best to let each couple interact with each other; do not break up the couples except for specific exercises when you and your co-therapist can go around and provide assistance to each couple separately. The strength of group therapy is largely in seeing others experience similar problems, hearing their suggestions, and experiencing their support. The therapist(s) should try to spend some time with each couple when all are role playing. If clients can model an appropriate behavior, the message is often better perceived and believed by the other couples than when the therapist does it. In addition, the couple doing the modeling experiences success, which is a positive incentive for further improvement.

EXECUTIVE SESSIONS

So far in this chapter, we have discussed the general communication process and have emphasized the nonverbal aspects of communication. Specific directions for teaching awareness and communication skills have been provided. Now, the training of the basic areas of marital communication will be described.

One of the most crucial skills in the communication process is listening. Many people who are called good conversationalists are essentially good listeners. Of course, talking and being articulate and expressive are important, but it is usually not there that the shoe pinches. Most people love to hear themselves talk and certainly do talk a lot when experiencing strong emotions. Since true communication is necessarily a two-way street, when a message is sent but not received communication is blunted.

Sometimes it is assumed that listening is a passive state. If this were true, listening would be easy and effortless. On the contrary, listening is a very active process indeed. Without exaggeration, one can speak of the *art* of listening. A good listener makes a very positive contribution to conversations and perhaps does more to keep the communication process going than the speaker. Effective communication also presupposes certain characteristics on the part of the listener. If we receive a message through a "filter" of our own—and the speaker may not even be aware of the existence of this screening device—we hear far more, or far less, than is actually said. Looking at the world through rose-colored glasses may create a pretty picture, but it is not reality.

To improve the client's ability to receive and send a message, the exercise called *executive session* has proved to be very helpful. An executive session can be defined as a planned, structured interaction in which partners take turns expressing their points of view, without interruptions, for a specified length of time and in a specific place. After one person has stated a brief one- to five-sentence message under the conditions described above, the listening partner repeats the essential ingredients of the message back to the speaker until the latter is satisfied that his/her message was accurately received. The first person then completes the process of interaction by acknowledging the completeness of the listener's feedback and, if necessary, by adding important elements that were not reported back.

Perhaps the most crucial characteristic of the executive session is its organization. Since this exercise aims at a gradual improvement of communication skills, it is systematic in its approach, setting specific behavioral limits and progressing from safe areas to more risky topics. The rather strict format of the executive session makes it far from spontaneous. Clients as well as therapists sometimes consider this a serious drawback; however, it should be remembered that we are dealing with the teaching and practicing of a particular skill and that each more advanced step is based on demonstrated competence lower in the communication hierarchy. The process is not unlike learning how to type, where the student starts with very prosaic finger movements in order to arrive slowly at the level where the skill has become automatic and spontaneous and all attention can be withdrawn from finger placements.

THE TOPIC OF THE EXECUTIVE SESSION

When clients arrive in the therapist's office, they have all too often reached the stage where a more than casual interchange easily escalates into a fight or where no meaningful communication takes place anymore. Usually, the couple has found that a certain set of topics is "safe" and can be brought up without fear of fights. Other topics are classified as explosive and are immediately thrown at one's partner when one feels attacked or embarrassed or when one wants to score a victory.

The eventual aim of the executive session is to help the couple freely discuss topics that were once invitations for insults and putdowns. The task for the therapist is to assist the couple in moving from discussing topics that divide the partners into two separate camps to discussing the same topics with mutual efforts at problem solving.

From our clinical experience we recommend that the following sequence be used in determining topics for the executive sessions:

1. Neutral topics
2. Positive topics
3. Requests for change
4. Sensitive and negative topics

Starting with a neutral topic is expedient, since even positive topics can provoke negative emotional reactions. The partners too easily can switch from positive conversation to argument or may conclude a positive statement with a barb or a criticism, such as "I really enjoyed it when we went out to dinner. We used to do that a lot when we were just married, but nowadays you always say that you don't have time or that it's too expensive," or: "You looked absolutely gorgeous when we went to that party last Saturday—why can't you fix yourself up like that all the time?"

Neutral topics may not contain much interest for the other partner, but that is no obstacle to learning the executive session format. Since we want the partners to practice a new skill and have to avoid moving too fast, a dull topic may be an excellent starter. The husband could describe his place of employment, a recent political event, an article he read in the newspaper; the wife could use similar topics or possibly talk about the traffic on her way to work, a popular television program, an incident that happened that day. If there's constant tension between the marriage partners, such a neutral topic will not increase that tension. For purposes of the executive session exercise in communication skills, one partner will then be able to state his/her message without interruption, and the other will be able to repeat easily the essential content of the message. This form of communication should be practiced several times before the couple is ready for the next stage.

— • —

When Arthur and Mary Peabody were ready to start their first executive session, their therapist assigned the astonished Arthur the task of describing the service station where he usually gets gasoline on his way to his office. His wife also was smiling surprisedly, but the result was a factual description of building, personnel, and street corner. Mary listened carefully and reflected back the description in great detail. Now the Peabodys understood the format, and the therapist assigned Mary the job of commenting on the way street-cleaning machines are built:

Therapist:	*That was very good, Arthur and Mary! Now let us reverse roles, with Mary as the speaker and you, Arthur, as the listener. Remember—no interruptions. Okay, Mary, describe to Arthur how street cleaners are built.*
Mary:	*Describe what?*
Arthur:	*You know, the street cleaners that . . .*
Therapist:	(Interrupting.) *It's Mary's turn to talk now, Arthur. I'm sure she knows what street cleaners are.*
Mary:	*Of course, but I was just surprised. OK, here we go. A street cleaner is a machine that looks like a tank. It*

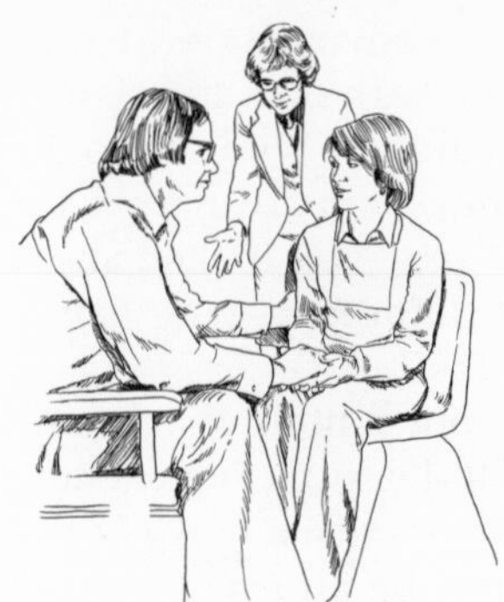

	has big brushes underneath and these turn around while water spurts out. The machine moves about five miles an hour and is usually used at night. That's about all, I guess.
Arthur:	*A street-cleaner is . . .*
Therapist:	(Interrupting.) *Remember, Arthur, you start by saying, "Mary, I heard you say that . . ."*
Arthur:	*You're right. OK, Mary, I heard you say that a street cleaner has big, rotating brushes that clean the street. Also, water is used. And . . . oh yeah, they go about five miles an hour, usually at night.*
Mary:	(Smiling.) *That's great, Art.*
Therapist:	*Was anything important left out?*
Mary:	*Not really, only that it looks like a tank.*
Arthur:	*You're right. I remember your saying that.*
Therapist:	*Both of you did a good job. You clearly know how to listen and report back. Let's try another one. Arthur, it's your turn. We have to make sure you both understand the process because there is an important homework assignment waiting.*

—— • ——

Although most couples will perceive the task as easy, you should provide ample training in the office to make sure that the format of the executive session is not only well understood but also smoothly executed. The in-office practice should be followed by precisely prescribed homework assignments for further practice during the week. Together with the therapist, the couple(s) should determine the place and time for their homework sessions and, if possible, the topics to be discussed.

GROUP THERAPY

If two therapists are working together, as is often the case in group marriage counseling, jointly they can demonstrate the desired behavioral format for the executive session. One therapist role-plays the speaker and the other therapist models the behavior of the listener, who reflects back the message. When group marital therapy is conducted by one professional person, the therapist role-plays being the speaker and each client, in turn, demonstrates an understanding of the listening and reflecting roles.

After all partners have practiced the reflecting role several times, the group therapist and the clients switch roles. Now each client assumes the speaker's role, behavior that has been modeled previously by the therapist. The client will find it easy to speak to the therapist, who then reflects back the message. All the marriage partners in the group practice the speaker role several times, while the therapist reflects the general content. Only when you are reasonably sure that your clients have acquired some competence as reflector and speaker should you have them start practicing both roles as a couple.

In teaching and coaching the executive session format, you should be active, guiding each partner with comments, such as "Be positive" and "Give praise," and guarding against pitfalls.

WIFE: Yesterday I went to the market and met Frank and Helen . . . you know, our neighbors who moved away last year. They told me that they have a nice four-bedroom house up north.

THERAPIST: *(Whispering a prompt to wife.)* Look at your husband . . . good.

WIFE: The house is not as big as the one they had here, but they have a larger yard.

HUSBAND: Why were they here?

THERAPIST: *(To husband.)* Hold it! Your task now is to reflect back. Save your questions for later.

HUSBAND: OK. You said that you met Frank and Helen yesterday in the market. They have a smaller house but a bigger yard.

THERAPIST: That sounds very good. *(To the wife.)* Was that all?

WIFE: Yes, I guess so.

THERAPIST: That was excellent. How do you two feel about communicating clearly?

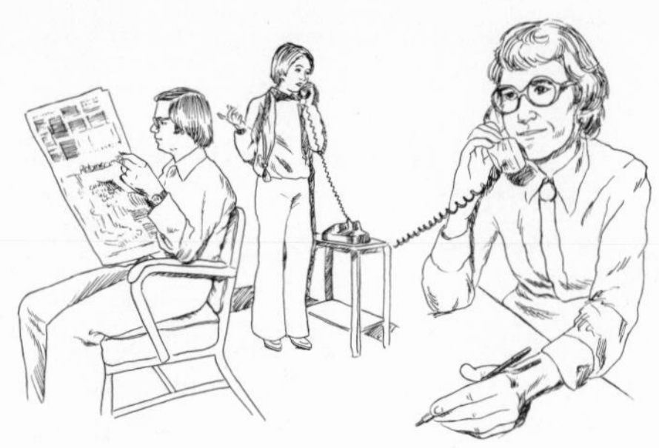

It may appear that caution is overemphasized here, but the aim is to have the couple practice executive sessions at home outside your influence. Overlearning is mandatory to guarantee success. After the correct behaviors have been acquired, the partners select two or three neutral topics for their executive sessions at home before the next therapy session. The topics should be determined in the therapist's office to ensure that neutral ones are chosen and to increase the commitment

TABLE II. Executive Session Report Form

Part 1 (to be filled out during the therapy session):

Name:

Spouse:

Place:

Time:

Topic:

Part 2 (to be filled out immediately after executive session):

Topic for discussion					
Place					
Time and date					
Duration					
	Excellent	Good	Average	Weak	Failure
My presentation					
Spouse's feedback					
Questions to ask therapist:					

to do the exercises at home. Forms are given to the clients to fill out when they have done their executive sessions at home. It is a good policy to request that the couple do an executive session two or three nights a week during the early stages of therapy. It may be necessary, with resistant clients, to phone them between sessions and to prompt and reinforce them to do the assignments.

At the beginning of the next therapy session, the clients report on the success of their executive sessions. They are to have filled out the "Executive Session Report Form" (see Table II) and are to bring one form along to the next appointment for each executive session held. A supply of these report forms can be found in the "Client's Workbook."

After therapist and clients are satisfied that the interactions over neutral topics are going smoothly, positive topics, then requests, and, finally, sensitive issues may be introduced. The same procedures as outlined above should be followed. You should make sure that the clients understand "positive topics" as messages containing compliments or other pleasure-evoking elements. Requests are just that: an expression of a desire to obtain something or to have the partner change something, but not a criticism! The sensitive topics include those elements that were reported as trouble spots in the marriage. Usually, you will have made a list of these items during the intake procedures, but additional items may have been added in the course of the therapy sessions.

Positive topics for Mary and Arthur Peabody included:

- Arthur is very accurate.
- Arthur is a neat dresser.
- Arthur maintains good relations with the neighbors.
- Mary is active in Lisa's school.
- Mary is working part time.
- Mary is a good mother to Lisa.

Requests for the Peabodys were:

- For Mary to make a special dessert
- For Arthur to water the yard
- For Mary to call Lisa, who is at a friend's
- For Arthur to select a given TV program
- For either one to join the other for a walk
- For either one to plan a weekend trip

Sensitive issues included:

- For Mary to clean the house
- For Arthur to express his feelings

- For Mary to work extra hours
- For Arthur to take care of Lisa
- For either one to discuss their financial future together
- For either one to discuss their sex lives

THE SETTING OF THE EXECUTIVE SESSION

In addition to the conditions regarding the topics for the executive sessions, attention should be given to a number of elements surrounding its setting. These include:

1. *Date.* Before the couple leave the therapist's office, they specify how often they will have an executive session before the next therapy meeting. In general, two or three per week work out well. To avoid overloading the couple with work, it is not advisable to have sessions each day. After the number of sessions has been determined, specific dates should be assigned for each session. Each partner fills out the appropriate dates on the "Executive Session Report Forms."
2. *Duration.* The couple decides in advance how long each executive session will last. From 5 to 10 minutes appears to be an appropriate length in most cases, but of course personal preference, the nature of the topics, and the progress and skill level of the clients should be taken into account. The therapist assists the clients in determining a specific manner in which to stop the conversation. Usually, verbal phrases will be used, such as "I'm feeling tired (or frustrated or uptight) now and I would like to stop our executive session now. Let's continue it tomorrow night at nine after the kids go to bed." Indicating a reason for stopping early is very beneficial; when a specific time is set for continuing, the spouse who wants to stop clearly indicates that there is no personal objection. Sometimes, signals function very well, since they do not interrupt the verbal interchange during the executive session. Satisfactory signals must be mutually understood and agreed upon, such as raising one's hand, crossing one's arms, or sitting back. When the partners agree to stop a specific session, they do not have to abandon the topic altogether. The conclusion of the executive session need not terminate the discussion of the issues and feelings.
3. *Time.* The couple should select a time that is mutually convenient. This time slot should be written on the appropriate "Executive Session Report Form" while the partners are still in your office. The time slot should be chosen in such a manner

that other duties or other people are not likely to intervene. For marriages with children, this often means that it may be wise to wait until the children have gone to sleep. A notoriously *bad* time is when one person is tired and is getting ready for bed.

4. *Place.* Along the lines of obtaining commitment and assuring success, a particular place for the executive sessions should be chosen and marked on the report forms. Inappropriate places include: at a cocktail party, in a car in heavy traffic, in front of a television set. It is helpful if the place selected suggests relaxation and intimacy, such as at the dinner table after the meal is finished or on the couch after a favorite television program is finished and the TV set is turned off.

——— • ———

INAPPROPRIATE PLACE/TIME

Husband: *Let's have the executive session.*
Wife: (Watching TV.) *Uh-huh.*
Husband: (After some time.) *Honey, it's getting late; we should start.*
Wife: *Oh, just wait till this TV program is over.*
Husband: *But I have to get up early.*
Wife: (No response.)
Husband: *Let's do it now; otherwise, I might as well go to bed.*
Wife: *We'll do it another time.*

APPROPRIATE PLACE/TIME

Wife: *The kids are in bed now and the place is quiet. Let's have our executive session now before your favorite TV program starts.*
Husband: *OK. And let's sit on the couch—it's nice and comfortable.*

APPROPRIATE PLACE/TIME

Mary and Arthur are sitting at the dinner table while Lisa is playing outside. Some of Arthur's favorite cherry pie is still on the table, and Mary has just poured a second cup of the expensive coffee Arthur has bought her as a surprise. They are looking at each other, seriously, but with twinkles in their eyes.

——— • ———

5. *Manner.* The partners should stick to the particular stage they have reached. Thus, when dealing with neutral topics, all emo-

tionally laden points are to be avoided. Similarly, once they have reached the stage of requests or sensitive elements, they should not hide in safe conversations but should trust each other and themselves. Feelings should then be expressed directly and each partner should own up to his/her emotions.

Here are two ways of dealing with a sensitive and charged issue, with one way leading to the problem-solving potential of an executive session.

—— • ——

INCORRECT, ACCUSATIVE RESPONSE

Arthur: (During an executive session at home while describing his office.) *And then there is Mrs. White—boy, is she a good worker, always on time and very accurate.*

Mary: (Interrupting.) *There we go again. Other people work hard and are neat, but your wife is a slob.*

Arthur: *Don't be so darned irritable. Besides, she is a lot better organized than you are. You sure could learn from her!*

By now, Arthur is pacing up and down the room, shouting. Mary has her head in her hands, pressing her temples. Upstairs, their daughter Lisa is listening with an expression of fear in her eyes.

CORRECTLY OWNING UP TO FEELINGS

The setting and topic are as described above. Arthur has described his office and has referred to Mrs. White. Mary has given accurate feedback and now proceeds to express her feelings about the topic.

Mary: *Arthur, when you told how neat Mrs. White was, I felt rejected. I felt that my work was criticized.*

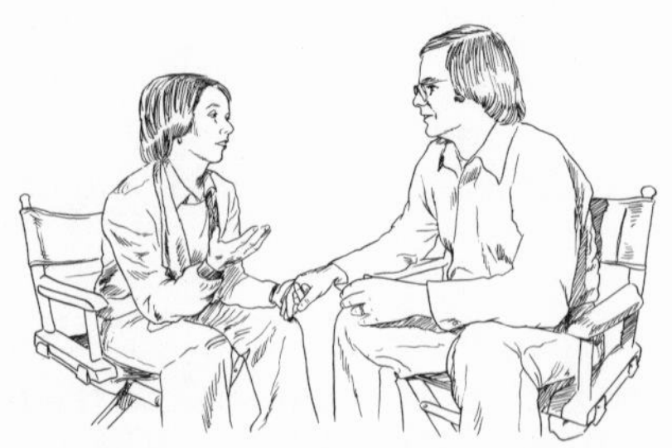

Arthur: *I didn't mean it that way, but perhaps we could make that a topic for our next session.*

Mary: *Sounds good to me. There's a lot there that is bothering both of us. Let me start by telling how I feel about my way of working, and you report back.*

Arthur: *OK, and then I would like to ask you something that is really important to me.*

Mary: *Sure. Now, I feel . . . etc.*

—— • ——

When practicing the more sensitive topics in the office, you might focus your clients' attention on the nonverbal behaviors expressed. These may, unconsciously or not, say more than the actual words spoken. Many people are more aware of picking up nonverbal meanings than of expressing them, and therapist's directing and modeling is often crucial. Let us not forget to be active and directive: we are dealing with people who have severe communication problems, and they need firm and specific guidance from an expert who is outside their relationship.

6. *Feedback.* During the practice in the office as well as when the clients report on their homework assignments, you should refrain from interpreting, intellectualizing, rationalizing, and other forms of verbal game-playing. Your clients need direction and modeling to acquire the correct behaviors, and the best way is to prompt, model, and provide positive feedback. Assignments and practice are crucial in acquiring a skill. Clients may understand the rationale of a behavior and still be unable to perform it. Therefore, you have to make sure to promote the correct approximations of the desired behavior. Settle for small improvements, a process of learning called *shaping*, and provide positive feedback for any sign of progress.

TYPES OF COMMUNICATION

To ensure that reciprocity remains positive in a marriage, various types of communication need to be taught to a couple. These forms of communication occur often in marital living, and your clients will need at least some training in all of them. Table III lists these communication skills. For each of these basic types of communication, the executive session format may be used both in the office and at home. Generally, each week a different type of communication may be intro-

TABLE III. Forms of Communication Skills Important in Marriage

1. Giving PLEASES.
2. Acknowledging PLEASES.
3. Asking for PLEASES.
4. Expressing *negatives.*
5. Exchanging physical affection.
6. Empathy.
7. Coping with unexpected hostility or persistent bad moods.

duced. It is important, however, not to pursue new types until the previous ones are understood and firmly ensconced in the couple's repertoire.

GIVING PLEASES

This may be the most obvious form of positive communication, and the clients will readily understand the need for exchanging pleasing behaviors. The marriage where no PLEASES are given is rare, since it could not last long! Unfortunately, PLEASES are frequently taken for granted or lack that personal touch or emphasis that makes them stand out as a ray of sunshine through a dark sky. Some examples of giving a PLEASE are:

- "That is a nice dress you're wearing."
- "I'll go to the store and get some of that special ice cream you like."
- "Let me take the trash out for you."
- "May I mix you a drink?"

You will find that most clients can come up with a good variety of pleasing behaviors, once they have learned to be attentive to them. The exercise called "Catch Your Spouse . . ." described in Chapter 4 can stimulate ideas for giving PLEASES.

ACKNOWLEDGING PLEASES

Many couples coming for marital therapy will lack skills here. Failure to acknowledge the everyday and ordinary positive things that are said and done is the main reason that once-satisfying marriages wind down and become lifeless exercises in which spouses take each other for granted. How many husbands comment favorably on evening meals prepared by their wives; and how many wives indicate that they appreciate the hard-working efforts of their husbands in earning the family living? It's easy to take the good things that go on in a marriage for granted.

You can highlight the importance of acknowledging PLEASES in a marital therapy group by going around to the members and asking them to recount a recent episode when their spouse did or said something nice but was not acknowledged for it. Usually, it is only necessary to have them focus on an event or interaction that occurred the same day of the session.

Joe, a druggist, was a man-about-town. He was active in local politics, ran for office on the town council, and participated in numerous organizations. He was particularly friendly and gregarious with the townspeople, who would come into his drug store for conversations each day.

However, he virtually ignored his wife, failing even to acknowledge her significant assistance and help to him as his bookkeeper and clerk in the store.

As you review each week's homework and progress, you should often ask whether pleasing talk and behavior was acknowledged to overtrain the spouses in the crucial skill.

THERAPIST: And, Linda, did John do something special for you this week?

LINDA: Oh, yes, he came home early last Friday and we went dancing. And on Sunday, we walked along the beach together.

THERAPIST: That sounds good to me. Did she thank you, John?

JOHN: She sure did! But then again, Linda always does.

THERAPIST: What did she do for you this week?

JOHN: Let's see—Sunday morning, she let me sleep in and made a special breakfast. Then Tuesday, we had apple pie, which is my favorite, and today she bought me a new set of golf balls.

THERAPIST: And did you thank her?

JOHN: No, I guess not, but she knows I appreciate it.

THERAPIST: Still, it's nice to hear it, isn't it, Linda?

LINDA: Yes, that's true.

THERAPIST: OK, John, tell her!

JOHN: OK, Linda . . . you know . . . uh . . . well, thanks for the pie and golf balls.

LINDA: You're quite welcome.

With a group of married couples, you can pair them up and ask each dyad to take turns acknowledging a PLEASE that has occurred in the past two days by using one of the pat phrases:

- "I like it when you do . . ."
- "It makes me feel good when you . . ."
- "Your saying that really helps."

Then, give them an assignment to use one of these reinforcing phrases each day during the next week when they "catch their spouse doing or saying something nice."

ASKING FOR PLEASES

Very often the skill of *asking for* PLEASES is missing in those marriages where the spouses are unhappy with each other. Both partners may assume that the other should know what is wanted or desired, as though spouses could read each other's minds. When the therapist suggests that it is important to request PLEASES from each other, a spouse is likely to object, stating, "My wife (or husband) should know what I want. After all, we've been married for umpteen years!"

Wives often find out that their husbands would be happy to assist with household chores or child-rearing responsibilities once they are given an affirmative request. Husbands, who believe that their wives would object to adding some variety to their sex life, are pleasantly surprised when they ask in a positive way for new sexual activities.

—— • ——

Dorothy, a 34-year-old mother of two children, was a teacher who had aspirations to attend graduate school for a master's degree in educational administration. She and her husband had agreed to limit their family to the two children but did not discuss birth control measures. She spoke with her gynecologist about having a laparoscopic tubal ligation (a simple surgical procedure that can be performed on an outpatient) after some of her friends had completed the procedure. She mentioned the idea to her husband in passing but chafed and felt hurt because he didn't spontaneously offer his encouragement and support. She was angry because he was so neutral about the procedure but didn't realize that she had failed to express directly to her husband how important his support and assistance would be to her.

—— • ——

Alice, a 46-year-old mother of three, simmered with anger and feelings of rejection for years because John, her husband, would characteristically walk a step or two ahead of her when they were out walking together. She finally began to grab him and request affirmatively that she wanted him to slow down and walk with her! She also learned, in therapy, how to ask John to help her with making plans for her senile mother.

—— • ——

Suppressing one's needs and wants leads to "gunnysacking," or simmering hostility and depression, and occasionally to emotional explosions, outbursts of acting out. It is essential to convince the marital partners that asserting one's needs is a constructive and positive contribution to the union. A chart that distinguishes passivity and aggressiveness from assertion, like that in Table IV, can sometimes clarify the concept and gain the couple's commitment to make requests of each other.

When the couple learn to ask for PLEASES directly, requests are more likely than not readily granted, and positive reciprocity builds up. For example, in the Peabody family, Arthur and Mary learned to ask for what each wanted from the other:

ARTHUR: Mary, this month, I have less hours at work than usual, but I still would like to put the usual $200 in our savings account. Could you stretch the budget an extra bit?

MARY: I certainly will try. Also, I might be able to put in some

TABLE IV. How Assertiveness Differs from Passivity and Aggressiveness on Behavioral Dimensions[a]

Passive person	*Assertive person*	*Aggressive person*
Has rights violated, is taken advantage of.	Protects his or her own rights and respects the rights of others.	Violates rights, takes advantage of others.
Does not achieve goals.	Achieves goals without hurting others.	May achieve goals at expense of others.
Feels frustrated, unhappy, hurt, and anxious.	Feels good about self, has appropriate confidence in self.	Is defensive and belligerent and humiliates and depreciates others.
Is inhibited and withdrawn.	Is sociable and emotionally expressive.	Is explosive, unpredictably hostile, and angry.
Allows others to choose for him or her.	Chooses for self.	Intrudes on others' choices.

[a]Adapted by James Teigen from *Your Perfect Right* by Alberti and Emmons (1974).

extra time myself at the job. Would you take care that Lisa does her homework when I work overtime?

ARTHUR: Sure. I should be with her more, anyway.

MARY: Yes, that would be good. Could you take her to the dentist tomorrow? Then I can check at the office for extra hours.

ARTHUR: OK, I'll take her tomorrow and drop you off on the way at the office—that saves gas. While you're at the office, would you see if you can get into a car pool? Even twice a week would make a big difference.

MARY: No problem. Karen will probably want to share the driving.

When spouses realize the existence of some unresolved issue, they can tell each other clearly and simply what they mean and especially what they feel. This direct expression of feelings is called *leveling*. It is important not to fall into the trap of accusing or blaming one's partner but to stick to one's own opinions and emotions. For example:

MARY: I'm going to the PTA meeting at Lisa's school tomorrow, Arthur. They're planning a sports day for the kids and want parents to help. I know you don't care much for that, but I still would like it very much if you would join me during some of the meetings.

ARTHUR: I'm sorry, Mary, but those meetings really get to me. I care about Lisa's work at school and I appreciate it that you go to the meetings, but they are too much for me.

MARY: I know you care about Lisa's work, Arthur, but I can't help feeling that you limit your involvement too much to academics. Lisa told me that she would like to see you at some events where the kids perform and, frankly, so would I.

ARTHUR: Maybe you're right. OK, I'll go to the play they'll be putting on, but I honestly don't want to get involved with the PTA.

MARY: That's fine, Arthur. I'm sure Lisa will like it when you come to the play, and I'm really happy that you'll join me.

In teaching a couple how to ask for their desires affirmatively, it is wise to demonstrate a few typical phrases that can be quickly learned and stored in memory:

- "I would like you to . . ."
- "It's very important to me that you help with the . . ."
- "It would make me feel better if you would . . ."
- "I'd appreciate your doing . . ."

These phrases can be practiced several times in the therapy session until they "feel" natural to the partners. Emphasize the importance of the nonverbal components in asserting desires: eye contact, volume and tone of voice, gestures, posture, and facial expression. The nonverbal dynamics should be consonant with what is said.

In doing marital therapy, we review the notion of "permission" with our couples. We ask each couple to discuss what they agree on for their relationship:

1. What do you ask permission of your spouse for?
   Examples: a major purchase, using a room for a new purpose, inviting the family to visit.
2. What decisions do you take for granted without asking your spouse for input?
   Examples: accepting certain types of invitations, making small purchases, preparing menus and food.
3. What do you reach a consensus on?
   Examples: moving to a new home, timing a pregnancy, deciding on a vacation.

One by-product of greater facility in making *I* statements that express one's desires is that both partners become more aware of their own and their spouse's values, hopes, wishes, and needs.

EXPRESSING NEGATIVES DIRECTLY

This is a difficult communication skill. Negative feelings include anger, hurt, disappointment, irritation, annoyance, rage, sadness, anxiety, depression, discomfort, and frustration. We call them *negative* not because they need to be intrinsically harmful but because of their colloquial association with unpleasant affect. We try to clarify for our couples in treatment that negative feelings are as important and natural in a marriage as positive feelings; their task is to express them in ways that produce constructive change in their relationship. The partners may have found that expressing negatives frequently results in fights because accusations multiply. You should present, demonstrate, and discuss the differences between direct, constructive expressions of "negative" feelings and indirect and hurtful expressions:

Appropriate	*Inappropriate*
Direct	Indirect
"Owning up" to one's feelings	Accusing the other person of something
Spontaneous	Delayed and "gunnysacking"
Expressing *now*	Withholding
Actively expressing	Passively withdrawing
Assertive	Sulking or aggressive
Describing the other's behavior	Interpreting the other's motivations

You might describe a formula for expressing negative feelings, even putting it on a blackboard or giving it to the couple as a handout. The formula includes three steps:

1. *Specify the behavior of your spouse* that has led to your "negative" feelings.
2. Describe and "own up" to your negative feelings.
3. Make a request that might improve the situation and your feelings by asking your spouse:
   a. To change words or actions in the present or the future
   b. For help in solving a problem or dilemma
   c. For time to reach a consensus, compromise, or clarification

Here are some examples of appropriate as opposed to inappropriate expressions of "negative" feelings. It may be instructive for your married clients to review examples like these to sharpen their ability to discriminate constructive from destructive anger and annoyance.

Appropriate	*Inappropriate*
"When you wear such old clothes to parties, it makes me feel bad about myself. I would feel better about myself if you would buy some new clothes."	"Why do you always dress like a shabby old man?"
"Playing the music so loud hurts my ears. Please turn the volume down."	"Don't you think the music is on too loud?"
"I get afraid when you drive so fast. Could you slow down?"	"How fast are you driving?"
"When you lie so still during lovemaking, it makes me feel rejected and turned off. What can we do to improve our sex?"	"You don't seem to be enjoying sex tonight."
"Raising your voice and shaking your fist at me only makes me scared. I can't say anything when I'm scared. Let's take ten minutes to cool off and then talk about it."	"You're a violent bully, just like your father was!"

When one spouse has some issue that is important to him/her but that is not resolved during the communication process, the topic will turn up again and again, often in indirect ways, thus forming a *hidden*

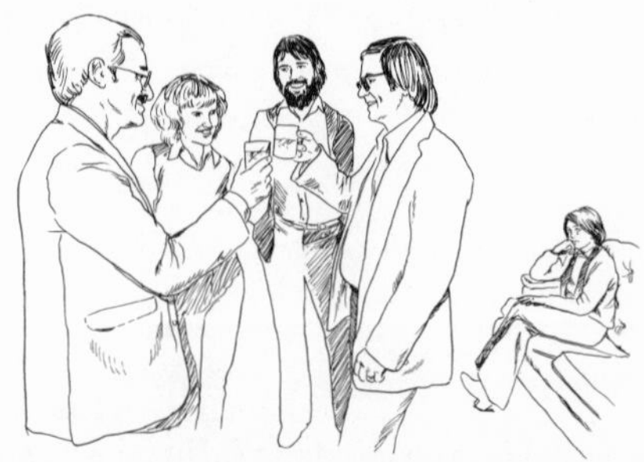

agenda. Not every topic can be discussed at any time. It is important to recognize the existence of a hidden agenda and to determine the best way of dealing with the issue.

As therapist, you will have to be active and directive in channeling each partner's "negative" feelings in a constructive way. For example:

THERAPIST: Sylvia, Bert did not thank you for washing the car. You didn't like that. Can you tell him this?
SYLVIA: I didn't like it when he did not thank me.
THERAPIST: OK, Sylvia. Turn to your husband, look at him, and say, "Bert, I did not like it when . . ."
SYLVIA: *(Looking directly at her husband.)* Bert, you did not thank me for washing the car and that made me feel bad. I felt taken for granted.
BERT: I am sorry. *(To therapist.)* She is so sensitive!
THERAPIST: Tell your wife!
BERT: Sylvia, you are always . . .
THERAPIST: *(Interrupting.)* No accusations, Bert! Tell Sylvia how *you* feel!
BERT: Sylvia, I sometimes forget things. I would like you to tell me because it is an honest mistake. Sometimes I have the feeling that you hold it all back and I feel caught in a storm of criticism all of a sudden.
SYLVIA: Thanks for telling me. I'll try.

There is a concept of *measured honesty* that can be used by married couples to guide them in deciding what and when to express in negative terms. Before communicating some negative feeling, a person should ask himself or herself:

- "Are my perceptions accurate?" (For example, "Did my husband actually make a pass at my friend?")
- "Can anything be done to change the situation that is producing my negative feelings?" (For example, "Should I tell my wife that I really prefer women with blue eyes and long legs while she has brown eyes and short legs?")
- "Is it necessary to express my feelings? Will I gain anything by it?" (For example, "Should I tell my husband that I had an unhappy affair ten years ago while he was stationed overseas?")
- "Is it timely to express my negative feelings?" (For example, "Shall I tell her that she hurt my feelings now at the party or shall I wait until we get home?")

Editing is an attitude of politeness of the spouses toward each other. When we know somebody else very well, we all too often ignore the common rules of courtesy. Our behavior toward close relatives is sometimes couched in words and actions that we would never dream of using with strangers. Polite behavior conveys respect—and intimacy is not a valid excuse for rudeness. In fact, recent research on marriages reveals that distressed couples tend to exchange negative feelings and hostility at a higher rate and more reciprocally than couples who are satisfied with their relationships. In other words, successful marital partners tend to let a certain amount of hostility go by without "getting back" at each other.

One couple, at the end of marital group therapy, spoke enthusiastically about how much help they had got from the group. Since they had hardly participated at all, they were asked in what way they'd been helped. The husband answered, "Every time we start to argue we say, 'Let's postpone this until the Wednesday night group meeting. We can bring it up for discussion then.' By Wednesday we've forgotten about it, and we find that most of our arguments have been trivial and unimportant. We use the methods we've learned to cope with important differences, but the frequency of arguments has gone way down!"

EMPATHY

When the clients learn to see the world through the eyes of their partners, communication becomes much easier. Empathy is difficult to learn, however, and you are advised to make ample use of feedback, doubling, and especially role reversal in teaching this skill during marital therapy. The executive session format is an excellent method for teaching empathy because each spouse has to reflect on what the other is saying and expressing. The role-reversal technique is most effective when the partners actually exchange seats. For example, using the episode described above, the therapist guides Bert and Sylvia through a role reversal to promote empathy.

THERAPIST: OK, Bert, sit in Sylvia's chair, and you, Sylvia, take Bert's chair. Good. Now, Sylvia, you play Bert and ask your wife to communicate her feelings more directly.

SYLVIA: *(As Bert.)* You should tell me how you feel.

THERAPIST: Express *your* feelings and make a request.

SYLVIA: *(Still as Bert.)* I feel lost when I don't know how you feel. Could you tell me when I do something that bugs you?

THERAPIST: Excellent!

BERT: Now I see what you mean.

SYLVIA: It seems so different when I say it!

THERAPIST: You look at it through Bert's eyes. Now, Bert, you be Sylvia and ask your husband to thank you for washing the car.

BERT: *(As Sylvia.)* I didn't mind washing the car, but I would like it if you would say you appreciate it!

SYLVIA: *(As herself.)* Actually, I *do* mind, but you helped me a lot this week, too. And I'm not even sure I thanked you!

THERAPIST: Very good. Now for some feedback: Bert, how did you feel being Sylvia?

BERT: I felt taken for granted doing something special and not being appreciated. I didn't realize what it meant to her; now I know.

THERAPIST: And you, Sylvia?

SYLVIA: I can see now that Bert did not forget on purpose and that it is OK for me to remind him directly how important a "thank you" is for me.

THERAPIST: We all learned a lot tonight!

While congruence and positive regard are important qualities that infuse successful relationships, empathy is particularly crucial in the intimate personal interaction of marriage (Rogers & Stevens, 1967). Empathy involves sensing the other person's "inner world of private personal meanings as if it were your own, but without ever losing the 'as if' quality." Empathy is essential to a growth-promoting marital relationship. The usual understanding marital partners give and receive is more of an evaluation from the outside. Husbands and wives tend to view each other in terms of their own "world" rather than opening up to the other's. Communicating the knowledge of what one's partner feels is only one part of empathy; the other part of empathy is the ability to experience what it *feels* like to be the other person. Putting both the cognitive and emotional components of empathy together for even occasional use in a marriage requires training and practice, even when the partners possess natural empathic skills.

Empathy, as a mutual exchange of feelings and information, can be taught to couples by using the executive session format. The executive session, in fact, builds in empathy as a communication exercise because it forces each partner to listen carefully, absorb the emotional and informational impact of the message, and check out the accuracy of her or his perception with the speaker. The executive session also has the effect of slowing down the communication process, thereby preempting the branching off into irrelevancies that can escalate into a brutal and hurtful exchange of anger.

— • —

In the following example, the therapist guides Ann and Jim into an empathic exchange by having them follow the executive session format.

Therapist: *Jim, you and Ann seem to be having some tension tonight over Ann's working hours. Let's put your thoughts and feelings out in the open through an executive session. Is that all right with you, Ann?*

Ann: *Sure. He's been steaming all night and I'm sure it's about my working overtime. But he doesn't say anything, he just glares at me.*

Therapist: *OK, then let's start by having you, Jim, tell Ann your thoughts and feelings about her working and Ann will listen carefully and repeat back to you what you've said before going on with her side of things.*

Jim: *Ann, it's just not fair to me and the kids for you to come home so late each night from work. I know you have a lot of responsibility at the office and that the doctors depend on you, but it's just not fair.*

Therapist: *Jim, that was a good starter. Can you also tell Ann how you feel when she comes home late?*

Jim: *Well, I guess it makes me feel jealous. I feel you care more about the doctors you work for than you do about me.*

Therapist: *Ann, it's your job now to reflect back to Jim what he's just communicated. Use your own words.*

Ann: *Jim, what I heard you say was that you feel jealous when I work overtime and that you don't think it's fair.*

Therapist: *Is that accurate Jim?*

Jim: *Yeah.*

Ann: *Well, we can't meet our expenses without my working and you know how hard it's been for me to find such a good job. Besides, I used to be very depressed staying at home and now I feel more confident and happy with this new job.*

Therapist: *Jim, can you repeat back to Ann what she's just said?*

Jim: *You said that we need the money from your job and that you're happier and more confident now that you have this job. Did I miss anything?*

Ann: *No. That's how I feel about it.*

Jim: *I really didn't know how important the job was to you. I figured you just didn't want to spend the whole evening with me, so I felt rejected.*

Ann: *You're saying that you were feeling rejected because I frequently have to work overtime and that you didn't know how important the job is to my self-confidence.*

Jim: *Right. Sometimes I even thought you might be having an affair with one of the doctors.*

Ann: *What!! How could you . . .* (interrupted by therapist.)

Therapist: *Wait a second, Ann. Don't run off on your own track until you've reflected back what Jim's just said. I know it's hard to listen to some things, but it's important in the executive session to respect each other's feelings and viewpoints enough to listen to each other before launching into your own feelings. So let's go back and reflect back what Jim just said.*

Ann: *That really threw me off base. I wasn't expecting that. Jim, did you say that you were thinking that I was having an affair with one of my bosses?*

Jim: *Well, what else could I think when you come home late without calling and always telling me how much extra work you have to do? I didn't realize that you enjoyed your job so much. I don't care for my job so much that I would willingly work overtime.*

Ann: *Let me assure you that I only have a business relationship with the doctors I work for. I respect them, but that's where it ends. In fact, I'd like to be able to tell them sometimes that I do mind so much overtime work. I can't seem to get the opportunity to tell them that I also have family responsibilities.*

The therapist can go on with Ann and Jim and help them further explore their feelings in the situation. Gradually, as they actively listen to each other's feelings, the therapist can coach them toward developing some alternative solutions to the problem and perhaps have Jim help Ann assert herself occasionally with her bosses so that she can more freely decide to work late or not depending on the situation. You can see how working on empathy brings into play all the other communication skills previously covered: giving and acknowledging PLEASES, *asking for* PLEASES, *and expressing negatives.*

—— • ——

Another way to help a couple build empathy is to have them write down their thoughts and feelings on a piece of paper. They should be instructed to write down anything that concerns them, whether it's about their feelings about work, their worries about the kids, or their anxieties in the relationship. After separately writing their lists, they are told to compare them and discuss their reactions. They will be surprised at how often they are unaware of or misconstrue what the other person is thinking or feeling.

Partners in distress have to learn, with the active coaching of a therapist, how not to interrupt each other, how to listen and hear each other through. The natural inclination of most spouses is to talk *at* each other, just waiting long enough to jump in with their side of the picture. Empathy takes time to establish as a regular way of communicating, but it is powerful nourishment for a relationship. Bringing even the smallest problems or most trivial feelings out into the open nullifies their destructive potential and makes it easier for partners to cooperate in changing the status quo. When communication between partners is free and direct, when there is a flow of feelings and ideas that are respected and heard, there can occur a special, exciting, and exhilarating experience of closeness and intimacy.

COPING WITH UNEXPECTED HOSTILITY AND PERSISTENT BAD MOODS

Once the couple experience a more effective and pleasurable way of communicating with each other, the unhappy past can be too soon forgotten. It may be quite a shock to encounter unexpected hostility, to experience persistent bad moods, or to find promises broken. Even after positive communication has been established, instances will arise where executive sessions or other coping skills are necessary to "detoxify" a situation. Some of these problem situations are:

1. Unexpected displacement of hostility, for example, from job to spouse, from children to spouse
2. Failure of spouse to comply with or fulfill a request or a promised course of action, for example, noncompliance with a specific agreement
3. Persistent anger and recriminations
4. Inexplicable bad moods, sulking, withdrawal

There are a variety of ways in which we've helped married couples cope with unexpected hostility, unprovoked anger, or unexplained irritability in their mates. No one coping method is guaranteed to work, so it is important that the couples learn a variety of methods and use one or more as needed to defuse the situation or alter its emotional tone in a more positive direction. We will take up each of the strategies for coping with hostility or unexplained bad moods, in turn; they are *ignoring, disarming with* PLEASES, *changing the subject to a mutual* PLEASE, *humor, repeated assertion, empathy, empathic assertion, time out,* and *positive greetings.*

Ignoring

One way to cope with unexpected and unjustified hostility is simply to ignore the outburst. In learning-theory terms, when ignoring some emotional behavior works and the behavior diminishes or stops, the process is called *extinction.* Ignoring can help to defuse a fight because it takes two to make a fight; however, it will not work if the emotional heat in one partner is so great that the ignoring actually serves as a further provocation. In such cases, ignoring can unfortunately fuel the fire and physical violence may ensue, so it is important to have the spouses learn to use their observation and intuition of how the ignoring is affecting the emotional partner, thereby determining when it is having desirable or undesirable effects.

One married woman who found this method to be helpful stated:

> "We're both very emotional people, but my husband is even more emotional than I am. And he will often be standing there, yelling about something that I really couldn't care less about. His yelling will have nothing to do with the problem at hand. And so I'll just retreat. I'll stand there and keep mixing up the pancake batter or whatever. Pretty soon he's standing there just sort of sputtering because I'm not giving him anything to respond to."

An old Spanish proverb sums up the coping skill of ignoring: "For a marriage to be peaceful, the husband should be deaf and the wife blind."

In teaching marital partners to ignore unprovoked anger or irritability, it is helpful for the therapist to point out repeatedly that the unpleasantness is not always aimed at the person who is the butt of the outburst. While a partner who is at the receiving end of nagging, argumentativeness, sulking, or hostility may feel as though the negative emotions are directed at him/her, most of the time they are not. Tell your clients that they should talk to themselves, telling themselves that they are not necessarily the target; they just happen to be there at the time. It is easier to maintain self-control and poise in the face of anger if you can tell yourself that what is bugging the other person belongs to him or her and not necessarily to the relationship.

Disarming with PLEASES

This method of coping is particularly helpful when a spouse is confronted with the early signs of unexplained irritability or disagreeableness in the partner. By responding with positive feelings, the partner's bad mood can be swept away and aborted before it gets in the way of the relationship. A good way to do this is by using nonverbal communication. A spouse can "melt" a bad mood by sitting next to the ill-humored partner, holding the partner's hand, rubbing the partner's neck, or giving a kiss or a warm hug. These nonverbal PLEASES, given in a free, spontaneous, and unsolicited manner, can overcome anger and irritability in a spouse just as they were often effective in the person's childhood when given by a caring parent.

— • —

One husband who frequently was irritable because of being preoccupied with work burdens and worries complained that he couldn't seem to change gears or move into a better frame of mind. These bad moods would occasionally lead into a fight. His wife learned to break through his bad mood barrier by giving him a foot or head massage, which relaxed him enough to "let go" without an explosion. Then, he was able to be with her in the here and now. He even began reciprocating in a similar way with massages when she had a bad mood.

— • —

Many couples report examples of having successfully used this approach; however, it is important to remind the couples you work with that this approach, or any other single approach, may not always work. It is vital that a range, or a combination, or a repertoire of coping responses be practiced and learned.

Changing the Subject to a Mutual PLEASE

This may be nothing more than suggesting to an aggravated partner that both go out for dinner, for an ice cream cone, for a cup of coffee at a restaurant, for a cocktail, or to a movie. Changing the scene helps to break up the stimuli that feed the hostility and annoyance, and moving into an activity that has been associated many times in the past with relaxation and pleasure helps to elicit positive feelings and thoughts.

— • —

Arthur: (Entering the house after a day at work.) *Boy, did I have a crummy day. I just feel like putting my fist through the wall. And why the hell didn't Lisa put her bicycle away? It's sprawled over the front steps!*

Mary: *Arthur, it's been a long day for me, too. Let's put the dinner I prepared in the refrigerator and go out to have a quick bite to eat and then see the new science fiction movie you were interested in.*

Arthur: *That sounds like a good idea. Let's get out of here before I blow my stack.*

Humor

Bringing up something totally incongruous, making a joke (even if it's a bad one), or clowning can change the emotional context from superserious to funny. Judy told the marital group how she gets her husband Bob through some bad moods by mimicking his pained facial expression. Her mimicry invariably brings a smile to his face and he takes himself and the situation less seriously. Another spouse said that when she lashes out at her husband for no good reason, he counters with mock hitting and mock name-calling that then lead to giggling and hugging.

Repeated Assertion

In this method, the spouse responds to unprovoked anger or crankiness by repeating, over and over again, a refusal to accept blame or share the partner's "suffering." In teaching this method to married couples, it is a good idea to have both partners agree to a "canned" statement that will be viewed in the future as a fair means of coping with unjustified hostility or irascibility. This method is sometimes called *the broken record* because the person reiterates the same statement, much as a broken record caught in a groove. The statements could be "I will not put up with being a target of your anger" or "I'm not going to spoil my evening just because you're in a bad mood." Again, the couples must be cautioned to try out this strategy and see how it affects the partner. If it backfires, obviously another strategy must be drawn upon.

Empathy

At times, the direct and accurate expression of empathy can be an effective means of coping with unexpected anger or moodiness. Extensive experience with the executive session format is necessary for empathy to have a useful role in crisis situations. When the spouses learn how to use reflection and clarification through empathy, they will slow down angry interchanges sufficiently to diminish the likelihood that escalation of destructive and hurtful aggression will occur.

— • —

If Arthur Peabody comes home irritable from a bad day at work and finds his wife Mary with a cold compress on her forehead in bed while the dinner (also cold!) is only half prepared, an altercation becomes likely. If Mary has learned to react with empathy, an escalation to a full-blown fight can be avoided. Arthur's remark "All day long I have been sweating in the office and now I also have to do the work here at home while you lie in bed!" can be countered by Mary with "I can see that it irritates you, Arthur. You had counted on a relaxing evening after a whole day at work." Arthur might still feel the need to add one or two criticial sentences, but Mary's empathy has probably set the scene for cooperation and communication, while a cutting counterattack would probably have led to a battle.

Similarly, Mary's being in a depressed state, complaining that her work at home is dull, meets with Arthur's empathic understanding if he says, "You found more satisfaction in your teaching career when we were just married, didn't you? How does substitute teaching look to you? Would you want to do it on a more regular basis? I could take Lisa to kindergarten on my way to work to make your morning hours more flexible."

Placing this in the framework of the executive session, Arthur could say, "Mary, I feel as if no one cares about my efforts at work when I come home and find dinner not ready. It seems as if I don't count at all." To which Mary can respond, "You feel unloved and not appreciated when dinner is not ready when you come home." Alternatively, if Mary expresses negative feelings, such as "Arthur, I feel put down when you criticize the way the house looks after I have been 'subbing' at school," an empathic response on the husband's part would be "Mary, you feel as if your work does not count when I complain about the house on the days you work at school."

—— • ——

Much practice and patience will be required before the clients have learned how to react to provocation and testiness with empathy, but they will soon discover that it reduces hostility and promotes positive communication. You will have little trouble convincing them of the value of empathy, but it will take a lot of coaching, modeling, and completed homework assignments to incorporate empathy in the marriage relationship.

Reflection, clarification, the sharing of meaning, and checking out accurate understanding are cornerstones in the building of genuine communication. Although the practice of these skills in your office may create an impression of artificiality, the saying that "Practice makes perfect" appears especially valid here and deserves the full commitment of both you and your clients.

Empathic Assertion

Sometimes, empathy alone is not effective, and it becomes necessary for the partner on the receiving end of unprovoked hostility to take a firmer stance. A combination of empathy and assertiveness is an alternative that couples can use with good results. Empathic assertion can be one of the most generally useful communication skills, not only with spouses but in many other casual and intimate relationships. In using it, a person begins by empathizing with the other and putting herself or himself in the other's position: "You seem to be really upset tonight" or "I can sense that you are very angry at me and the kids." Next, the assertive phrase is expressed so that the person clearly indicates an affirmative and constructive stance: "You seem to be really upset tonight, but I still want to discuss our plans for the weekend" or "I can sense that you are very angry at me and the kids, but your anger is coming from someplace else and we're not going to take responsibility for it." Usually, empathic assertion ends with a request for a change in the petulant spouse's behavior, for a compromise, for a discussion to resolve the problem, or for a request to use a time out.

Time Out

One way of coping with hostility is to allow oneself sufficient time apart to absorb the hostility, to let it decline in intensity, and then to express one's feelings in an assertive, nonjudgmental manner. Putting space between yourself and your spouse when negative feelings are in the air is called *taking a time out*. In fact, recent research indicates that satisfying marriages are distinguished from distressed ones by the lack of retaliation or reciprocity in the expression of negative feelings. Thus, *time out* and *ignoring* may be critical skills for marital satisfaction.

—— • ——

Arthur: (Coming home.) *This whole house is a mess again. I almost broke my neck over the vacuum cleaner and now I can't even sit in my own chair because you've got clothes all over the place!*

Mary: (Who had been busy cleaning the linen closet.) *Arthur, I was doing . . .*

Arthur: (Interrupting.) *Doing what? Here I work all day and you can't even keep this damn house in order.*

Mary: *Arthur, I see that you are angry, and I feel I am getting angry, too. I don't want to get into an argument now. Therefore, I'm going to the store now—I'll be back in half an hour. We'll talk then if you want.*

This cooling-off technique, called *time out* from anger-provoking situations, is highly recommended. However, in explaining time out to your clients, be sure to stress that the spouse who leaves must tell the other spouse where he/she is going and when he/she will be back. The spouse taking a time out should not leave in anger. Time out provides both parties with a space and a time for a cooling-off period.

—— • ——

Arthur: (When Mary comes back.) *I am sorry. I shouldn't yell at you, but I got a ticket coming home and it wasn't even all my fault.*

Mary: *Your criticizing me really made me feel bad. I was trying hard to do what you have asked me to and straighten out the whole linen closet, only to find you angry. But now I understand how you came to be angry, so we'll take it from here.*

Arthur: *Let me help you put the things back into the closet.*

—— • ——

Carefully outline the steps of using the time-out procedure so your couples in therapy will use it effectively. Each partner should be able to use time out correctly by:

1. Specifying the behavior in the other that is causing a problem ("When you shout at me for no good reason . . ."; "When you are silent and withdrawn for hours on end . . .").
2. Expressing her or his own feelings in reaction to the hostility or ill temper ("When you shout at me for no good reason, it makes me feel scared and uptight"; "When you are silent and withdrawn for hours on end, it makes me feel irritable and guilty").
3. Explaining the reason for the time out ("So I'm going to take a walk to try to collect my feelings").
4. Indicating how long the time out will be ("I'll be back in thirty minutes").
5. Saying where she or he will be ("I'm going to walk to the store").
6. Stating that he or she will be glad to talk about the situation on returning ("I hope we can talk about your feelings and what's bothering you when I get back").

Positive Greetings

First impressions are often decisive when a couple meet after being apart for most of the day, so greeting skills are crucial. You may want to work on greeting techniques, that is, teaching couples constructive ways of greeting each other when they come together at the end of a day can circumvent and prevent blasts of unexpected irritation or unexplained moodiness. These negative emotions are all too often taken personally by the receiving spouse, even though the source of the upset comes from elsewhere.

Consider how the therapist deals with the following situations that arise when Arthur Peabody comes home:

Mary: *I have had a headache all afternoon!*
Therapist: *Don't surprise him with a complaint. Can you start with a supportive question, like "How was your day?"*

Mary: *The bill for the car insurance came.*
Therapist: *Don't hit him where it hurts most. Can you rephrase that into something like "Oh, Honey, I'm glad we could save something extra last month because we will have the extra burden of insurance this round." And, even then, it's better to wait until after dinner to mention the insurance bill.*

Mary: *I am going to bed. Supper is in the oven!*
Therapist: *Help Arthur understand that you do not feel well and that you regret not being able to have dinner with him.*

Arthur: *Is dinner ready?*
Therapist: *Show Mary that you care about her and that you appreciate the extra effort she puts into the housework.*

Arthur: *Lisa, turn off the TV and do your homework.*
Therapist: *Mary is already afraid that your relationship with Lisa is a bit strained. Can you ask Lisa first what she is watching and then ask her if she has finished her assignments?*

These and similar situations are excellent opportunities for role-playing more positive alternatives that can lead to problem solving. You should have the clients go through a series of greetings and good-byes so that they experience the differences between positive and negative interactions. Feedback, coaching, prompting, modeling, and role reversal are again highly recommended techniques. Even when you model the appropriate behavior, the client may not always imitate it correctly.

—— • ——

Arthur: *Mary, is dinner ready? I'm late already.*

Therapist: (Modeling for Arthur.) *Mary, I don't want to rush you, but I am really pressed for time. Could you serve dinner early today?*

Arthur: *I'm pressed for time, Mary. Can I have dinner right away?*

Therapist: (Modeling again for Arthur.) *Mary, I don't want to rush you, but I have to be at the college early today for a meeting. May I help by setting the table?*

Arthur: (To the therapist.) *Oh, come on, now! You're overdoing it.*

Therapist: *You want to have dinner early, don't you?*

Arthur: *Okay, you're right. Mary, I'm sorry if I seem to rush you, but the college called an unexpected meeting. Do you mind if I eat as soon as you are ready?*

EXCHANGE OF PHYSICAL AFFECTION

Many couples have difficulty in physically expressing warmth and feelings of intimacy. A hug, a kiss, and a light caress of the neck or the ear are recognized by many people as expressions of endearment and caring. They are seen by many as communications that are pleasurable to give and receive. Unfortunately, when the romance and honeymoon are over, too many couples forget this powerful means of positive communication. For example, husbands often complain that their wives do not hug, kiss, or cuddle enough, and many wives complain that their attempts to cuddle, hold hands, or kiss their husbands are not interpreted as signs of affection but rather as sexual overtures. One goal of communication training is to help couples learn how to express their affection for one another physically. To reach this goal, couples need to learn how to ask for physical pleasure and to give appropriate verbal and nonverbal feedback during physical contact. Partners who freely give pleasure, ask for pleasure, and provide feedback on physical affection are emotionally aware of each other's feelings and will more frequently express feelings of warmth and intimacy. Teaching a couple how to express physical affection should be preceded by their first learning how to give PLEASES, ask for PLEASES, and give positive and negative feedback effectively.

Perhaps more than in any of the other communication training areas, it is important to introduce the couple to physical communication so that favorable expectations are raised. Your orientation should convince the couple that by acquiring these skills they can enhance their relationship. You might start your orientation by discussing how all human beings have an innate need for physical touching and closeness. When infants are deprived of physical touching and fondling, they can die. In adults, the lack of physical contact may lead to feelings of loneliness and isolation.

Couples can learn to communicate physically through a series of exercises and homework assignments. As with the other communication skills discussed in this manual, the sequence in which the exercises are used with couples experiencing difficulty in their relationship is very important. The initial exercises involve nonsexual parts of the body and are implemented under the supervision of the therapist, and later exercises involve homework assignments that may culminate in sexual intimacy.

HAND CARESS EXERCISE

The first exercise is a hand caress. In order to overcome self-consciousness and set a light tone for the hand caress, a warm-up exercise called "thumb talk" is helpful. Instruct the couple to cup their right hands slightly, interlock their fingers and point their thumbs up. Have the couple pretend that their thumbs are old friends who haven't seen one another for a long time and show how they might greet each other (without words, obviously, since thumbs don't talk). Now, show how they might fight. Have them make up. Show them loving and caring. Ask the couple if they enjoyed this, and emphasize that learning to communicate without words can be enjoyable and fun. Point out that a great deal of information about one's feelings can be conveyed through even simple physical communication.

After the thumb talk warm-up, you can start the hand caress exercise by first demonstrating a variety of caressing techniques. You can do this with a co-therapist or with one of the marital partners if you are the sole therapist. During the demonstration, the couple's attention should be directed to how the therapist initiates requests for physical stimulation and gives instructive feedback to help guide the person who is doing the massage. After the modeling by the therapist, the partners should take turns initiating requests and giving feedback. The

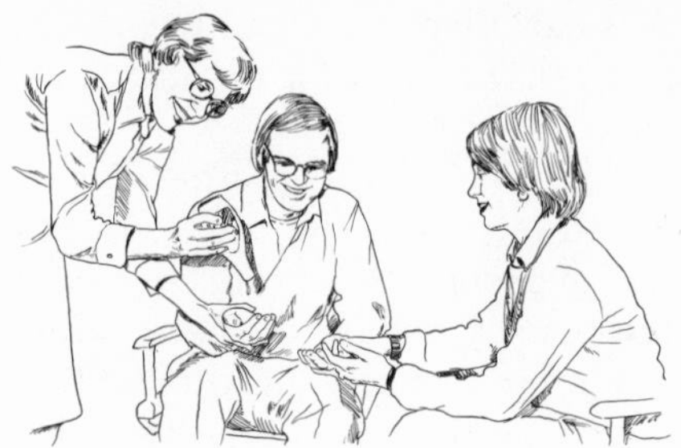

therapist can highlight the learning process by pointing out both appropriate and inappropriate ways of verbally communicating desires to one another.

Examples of inappropriate communication are:

- "You are pressing too hard. Why are you so clumsy?"
- "Can't you be more gentle?"
- "Joe told me about the fantastic massages his wife gives him."
- "It's too bad your hands are not as strong as Bill's. He could really rub me the right way!"

Examples of appropriate communication are:

- "I would love it if you could give me a massage."
- "Please go easy on my hand. It feels better when you stroke it lightly."
- "I really like it when you rub my hand lightly and slowly. It makes me feel close to you."

In setting up the hand caress exercise, instruct the couple to face each other and instruct one of them to take the other's hands. Pass out oil, lotion, or powder and observe and monitor the couple's efforts in initiating and giving feedback as they alternate caressing each other's hands. You should use prompts and feedback liberally to shape and mold appropriate verbal exchanges. The hand caress exercise should be completed after each spouse has received and given three to five minutes to hand caressing. After the exercise is completed, prompt the couple to share their experiences and feelings. You might ask, "What did you like about this exercise?" or "What kind of positive feelings developed from having your hand caressed?" The couple may then follow their positive feedback by making one or two behaviorally specific suggestions for improvement if the exercise needs to be repeated.

REQUESTING SEX

One form of physical expression that couples often have a great deal of difficulty with is asking for sex. Since any form of physical caress may be misinterpreted as an indication of sexual desire, it is important that the couple practice expressing their desires verbally as well as physically to discriminate physical indications of warmth, endearment, and intimacy from sexual overtures. Additionally, both partners typically need to learn ways of declining sexual requests in direct, honest, positive ways that will maintain feelings of intimacy and caring while indicating that now is not the time.

—— • ——

Requests for sex need not always be in the form of words. At this point in a marital group, one wife told the assembled couples that she and her husband had worked out a reliable signal that served to communicate her desire for sex. The signal was her donning an especially seductive nightgown. Such nonverbal signals for sex can be effective, but it is important to inquire if and how they are being used. A seductive nightgown will not elicit sexual intimacy if it is always kept at the bottom of the dresser drawer!

—— • ——

The issue of spontaneity often comes up in discussions of sexual interaction during marital therapy. Typically, husbands will want greater spontaneity in the decision to have sex and wives will want more advance notice. This distinction correlates with the generally accepted observation that men's sexual arousal is more rapid and under less stimulus control than women's. Women need more time to "get in the mood" and to have foreplay before being ready for sex. One couple we worked with arrived at a compromise between the husband's desire for immediacy and the wife's desire for gradualness in their sex life. They agreed to the husband's giving his wife at least an hour's advance notice of his interest in sex except for one night each week when he could initiate sexual advances on the spot. They referred to the spontaneous evening as the husband's wild-card night and used it effectively. It is important to note, however, that the compromise was worked out after the couple had acquired considerable skill in communicating their desires and in active listening and empathy.

The sex request exercise can be introduced by briefly explaining the above rationale. The therapist then alternately models appropriate (direct, clear, and positive) ways of asking for sex and inappropriate (indirect, vague, and demanding) ways of asking for sex. Attention is given to making the verbal and nonverbal dimensions of the request congruent.

Examples of inappropriate requests for sex are:

- "I suppose you're not in the mood?"
- "Do you have a headache tonight?"
- "You haven't been in the mood for three weeks now—do you think you might be up to it tonight?"
- "How come I *always* have to initiate our getting together?"

Examples of appropriate requests for sex are:

- "Let's make love tonight."
- "I'd like for us to turn off the TV, pour some wine, and go into the bedroom for some 'fooling around.'"
- "I'm in the mood for love and would like for us to reserve some time for each other before we go to bed tonight."
- "I'd really like it if you'd give me a slow and tender massage before we have sex tonight."

The couple should then take turns role-playing asking for sex. Instruct the partner who is receiving the request to respond verbally in a positive manner. As the therapist, you should use prompts and feedback liberally to shape appropriate verbal exchanges. Timing is an important dimension in making successful requests for sex; thus, orient the partners to tune in to the other's mood and to the existence of distractions. Make sure that the messages are specific and that they contain a feeling component. The partner who received the request can also be called on to give specific positive feedback and constructive suggestions for alternative forms of requests.

After each partner has mastered asking for sex in an appropriate manner, you should model declining a request for sex in appropriate and inappropriate ways.

Examples of inappropriate ways to decline sex are:

- "You have a one-track mind."
- "Why are you such an animal?"
- "I've told you a hundred times, I'll initiate our lovemaking when I'm in the mood."
- "Your timing is bad."

Examples of appropriate ways to decline sex are:

- "I'm glad that you want to make love with me this evening, but I'm really not in the mood right now. Perhaps we could just cuddle for a while and have sex in the morning."

- "It makes me feel good that you're attracted to me physically, but I've had a rough day and don't think I could really enjoy sex right now—how about tomorrow?"

The couple should then take turns role-playing asking for sex and declining that request in an appropriate manner. Again, you should use prompts and feedback to shape appropriate verbal and nonverbal exchanges. After the couple have practiced making and declining sexual requests and they feel somewhat comfortable with one or two alternatives, this exercise can be ended.

HOMEWORK ASSIGNMENTS

At the conclusion of these brief exercises, most couples are in need of further practice in the physical expression of warmth and feelings of intimacy. Furthermore, our goal is to increase the frequency of these appropriate expressions in the couples' everyday lives. Therefore, a homework assignment should be made. The homework assignment has three components:

1. Asking for some physical affection:
   "I'd love a kiss from you right now."
   "I'd really appreciate it if you'd give me a back massage."
   "I'd like you to hold me close and cuddle me while we watch this old movie."
2. Giving appropriate verbal feedback during physical affection:
   "When you kiss me like that, I feel like a million dollars."
   "I'm really enjoying this massage. Please rub a little lower and slower."
3. Specifying the time, place, and frequency for this expression of physical affection to occur.

We have found that couples need to practice requests for low-intensity, casual affection at least five times each day. Requests for casual affection include such things as asking for a hug or a kiss. If these types of quick-and-easy affectionate exchanges can be increased in frequency on a regular and spontaneous basis, then the rising level of reciprocity engendered will markedly improve marital satisfaction. The couple should also practice requests for sex two or three times during the week if the likelihood of their successful completion is good.

The homework assignments need to be individualized and tailored to the sociocultural and personal style of each partner. Each partner should decide on a physical request that is personally meaningful. If the couples cannot think of some physical requests on their own, you may want to suggest some of the following requests:

- Holding hands
- Taking a walk with arms around each other's waists
- Giving a hug
- Giving a kiss
- Giving a hand, foot, or face massage
- Brushing, combing, or washing the partner's hair
- Taking a shower or bath together and washing all over with soap
- Holding and caressing the partner's body
- Caressing the sexual organs
- Having sex

While relatively simple problems in sexual communication, such as the ones described above, can be effectively managed in marital therapy, more long-standing or complicated problems should be dealt with in behavioral forms of sexual therapy. These problems include primary nonorgasmic deficits in women, dyspareunia, severe premature ejaculation, impotence, and chronic cases of sexual disinterest and nonarousal.

If you have the skills to conduct more elaborate courses of sex therapy, you can help a couple with their sexual problems as you conduct the more comprehensive marital therapy, too. However, since sex therapy has become a subspecialty of its own within the helping professions, you may elect to refer your clients to more experienced sex therapists. Workshops, seminars, audiotape cassettes, and books are available to upgrade your skills in the sexual arena of marital therapy.

Additional references on sex therapy that can serve the marital therapist as specialized resources in helping married couples improve or enrich their sexual interactions are listed at the end of this chapter.

NEGATIVE FEELINGS

In the previous section of this chapter, we discussed six types of communication within the framework of positive reciprocity. Dealing with negative feelings and the expression of empathy often presents the greatest difficulty, and therefore, these modes of communication are discussed in greater detail in the rest of this chapter.

Executive sessions dealing with neutral and positive topics will have improved the couple's communication skills, but the transition to negative feelings is difficult. As the therapist, you face the problem of establishing in the couple the conviction that negative emotions are not necessarily expressed to hurt each other. On the contrary, appropriately expressed negative feelings do not contain accusation or aggression; they convey one's own hurt rather than inflicting hurt.

When dealing with negatives, you may want to spend some time exploring the breadth of this area without giving the couple opportunities for making destructive complaints about each other. Negative feelings and their proper expression are as much a part of a healthy relationship as positive feelings. Common negatives include anger, hurt, annoyance, jealousy, frustration, and disagreement. Then, there are the less aggressive but frequently more penetrating negative feelings of sadness, hurt, grief, and loneliness. At this stage of therapy, the emphasis is not placed on catharsis or ventilation of feelings. That opportunity was provided during the initial evaluation sessions. Now, the task for the couple is to learn how to deal with negative emotions, how to express them in constructive ways so that the marital relationship is strengthened, not undermined.

Some books have been published that can help married couples discriminate between destructive and constructive methods of expressing negative feelings. You should keep in mind, however, that simply referring a client to a book will not ensure that the material will be read or assimilated. You should consider setting aside a little time in each session to review and quiz the couple on their "bibliotherapy" if you decide to give readings as homework. Additional references for couples who might benefit from reading about the expression of negative feelings can be found at the end of this chapter.

Below are a series of guidelines that you can use to clarify the distinction between appropriate and inappropriate ways of expressing negative emotions.

EXPRESS FEELINGS DIRECTLY

Vague, indirect words do not touch the real issue but leave a bitter aftertaste. It is correct to own up to feeling hurt because one's partner forgot the wedding anniversary, but it is not correct to beat around the bush, hinting that feelings are hurt without coming out and stating this explicitly. Indirect communication does not fully release anger and tension, and, therefore, one may later add something extra and out of proportion to the scene of action. At the same time, indirect statements prevent the receiving party from making a clear counterexchange and moving toward problem solving. It is common for indirect communications to consist of short statements that get progressively more pointed and more irritating, finally resulting in a full-blown fight. Here is an example of how indirect expressions of negative feelings can escalate into a bitter fight that no one wins.

Husband:	(Coming home from work.) *It was a bad day at work—John forgot some of the tools and we lost two hours driving up and down.*
Wife:	*I'm glad that you don't forget important things.*
Husband:	*What do you mean?*
Wife:	*Oh, nothing.*
Husband:	*Don't give me that! What's the matter?*
Wife:	*It's not important—anyway, not to you—obviously.*
Husband:	*For heaven's sake, don't play those sulking games with me. I'm not one of your coffee-drinking, gossiping friends.*
Wife:	*What's wrong with my friends? At least they don't forget their wedding anniversary.*
Husband:	*Oh, is that all?*
Wife:	*Is that all? Is that all? You think only of your work, and, oh, yes, you also know the scores of all the baseball games.*
Husband:	*Women! Forget it! I'm going to the bar!*
Wife:	*Sure, live it up while I slave away all day long!*

A completely different situation could have been created if the wife had said, "I really felt sad and hurt when you forgot our anniversary. That day means a lot to me because you mean a lot to me."

OWN UP TO YOUR OWN FEELINGS

It is appropriate for spouses to *own up* to their feelings, but not to *accuse* each other of something. Apart from the fact that accusations rarely produce desired improvements in the other person, they tend to fuel fires beyond the immediate topic and the dragging of old skeletons out of the closet. Accusations, even subtly made, tend to reincarnate old battles and reopen old wounds from the past. Blaming or calling a name makes empathic acknowledgment from the partner almost impossible. Nothing remains to do but make a counterattack or a withdrawal into silence. Telling one's partner that "I feel bad and embarrassed about your excessive drinking at the party" is constructive and will hopefully elicit feelings of regret. On the other hand, a pronouncement that "You are an inconsiderate and tactless drunk whose only interest is the bottle and who always makes a complete fool of himself" is not very likely to meet with expressions of remorse.

EXPRESS FEELINGS WHEN THEY OCCUR

Spouses usually get angry when their feelings are hurt. When anger or other hurt feelings are allowed to simmer, without immediate expression, they can grow and become transformed into guilt, feelings of worthlessness, and depression. Bad feelings kept inside for too long can later blow up out of proportion to the original cause. Holding in negative feelings also takes effort and preoccupation, leaving less energy for expressing positive feelings.

Usually, negative feelings are communicated most effectively when done spontaneously. This does not mean they should be expressed in a fit of anger. The choice of place and time, and certainly the choice of words, is crucial; some lapse of time between the offensive act and the expression of the negative reactions evoked by it may be necessary. However, delaying the expression of hurt feelings increases the hurt and makes future release much more difficult. The building up of negative feelings can lead to gunnysacking, that is, storing up grievances and annoyances over a period of time and then keeping them ready for use against one's spouse later. Accumulating anger and bitterness by letting bad feelings simmer in one's gunnysack instead of expressing them directly and honestly when they actually occur will increase distress and dissatisfaction in a marriage.

When gunnysacking is a preferred mode of operation, the old wounds are deliberately kept open. The person will be inclined to periodically review the list of hurts and guard them almost jealously. No change of offensive behavior is sought; rather, one is on the lookout in order to collect further evidence to justify one's anger. Appropriate expressions of negative feelings include spontaneously and immediately telling one's partner:

- "It makes me feel overburdened and abandoned when you don't help with the daily chores."
- "I feel so alone when all the household errands and bills fall completely on my shoulders."
- "Having to take care of the children totally by myself makes me feel tired and constantly rushed."

BE ASSERTIVE, NOT PASSIVE OR AGGRESSIVE

Passively withdrawing rarely reduces feelings of tenseness and anger. If one can express clearly and actively what caused the hurt and what conditions are producing tension, the chances of obtaining relief are greatly increased. Assertive expressions involve pointing to some

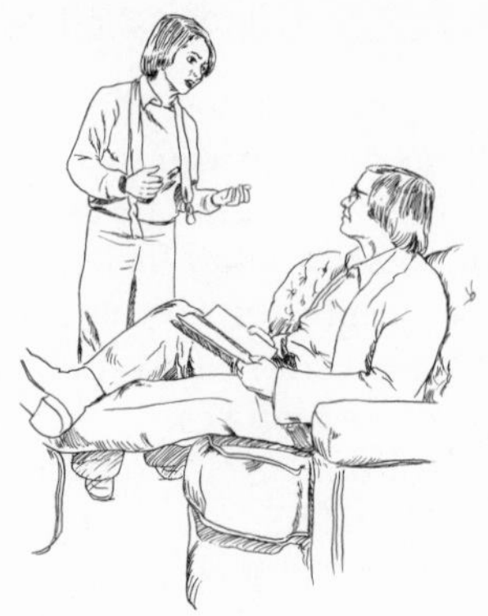

specific actions of the other person and describing how those actions produced bad feelings. Such direct expressions of self-assertion will be more readily received and listened to by a partner than his or her having to infer from passive withdrawal that something bad or negative is felt.

Here is an example of our couple, Mary and Arthur Peabody, expressing feelings directly and assertively to each other:

Mary: *Arthur, there is something I'd like to talk to you about for a moment. Are you in a rush?*

Arthur: (Putting his paper away and sitting back.) *No, I have plenty of time.*

Mary: *Okay. You know, it really bothers me when you talk harshly to Lisa. I know that she needs discipline, and she was really wrong in lying as she did yesterday.*

Arthur: *We can't let that pass.*

Mary: *No, I agree. But I felt that Lisa was almost terrified when you raised your voice so loud, and hitting her was not necessary, I feel. That makes me feel that the rule becomes more important than the person. I feel ill at ease when you do that. It really upsets me, too. I know that you love Lisa and that you want the best for her, but could you try to be less rough on her?*

Arthur: *I guess you're right. I don't go for lying, and I definitely want to put a stop to it, but I don't want to scare Lisa away from me. And I certainly don't want to upset my wife!*

Mary: *Thanks, Arthur. I know you care.*

Make sure your clients understand the differences between passivity, assertiveness, and aggression, which are outlined in Table IV on page 115. Here is an example of a passive response from a husband in a situation that calls out for assertion on his part.

—— • ——

Wife: *You're late again! I get fed up waiting with dinner—the kids and I ate already.*
Husband: *I'm sorry.*
Wife: *You can find food in the oven. Everyday you have some other excuse!*
Husband: *I can't help it . . .*
Wife: (Interrupting.) *You make sure you are in time for work in the morning. It should be possible to make it back in time.*
Husband: (No response.)
Wife: *You don't care about your family. I'm just a maid here. But at work it's, "Yes, Sir," "No, Ma'am."*
Husband: (Goes off to the kitchen.)

—— • ——

Closely related to passive withdrawal are inappropriate sulking and indirect or passive aggression. Here again, the negative emotions are not vented but the anger and hurt are kept alive. Both aggression and passivity are extremes and usually provoke more negative reactions. On the other hand, if one can be assertive by directly expressing the feelings of hurt or anger evoked by the insulting statement or inconsiderate action of the other, real communication becomes possible and both partners can attempt to see the other's point of view, as in the next example:

—— • ——

Wife: *Pete, it really upsets me when you come home so late.*
Husband: *I'm sorry, Connie. We had an unexpected emergency at work and the traffic was bad.*
Connie: *I still feel very upset, Pete. I know that you are punctual at work and when you come home late so often, I feel unimportant, as if work comes first.*
Pete: *The job is important to me, Connie, but you know that the family comes first.*
Connie: *I know. I didn't mean it that way. But can't you ask to get out half an hour earlier?*
Pete: *I'm afraid that's impossible, but I can ask to be*

assigned calls closer to home toward the end of the day. Then I can come directly here afterwards and avoid the traffic.

Connie: *That would really make me happy!*

Pete: *I'll talk to the boss tomorrow. He won't like it, but I know he wants to keep me. And the firm can afford to let me drive the truck home in the evening.*

—— • ——

Before actually having the couple try an exchange of negative feelings, it is advisable for you to model the action. If you are working with another therapist, the two of you should simulate a marital dyad, model the appropriate and the inappropriate behavior consecutively, and then ask the clients for reactions. As you model the inappropriate way of expressing negatives, we advise you to exaggerate deliberately, as this has a double advantage: it avoids rekindling the old fire since each partner knows "This is not me!" and it demonstrates what triggers or increases a conflict. Enlisting client reactions to these modeled scenes is an effective teaching device. Their reactions to the modeling will provide a sense of security to the spouses as they anticipate role playing themselves. They can detect what behavior is wrong, so chances are that their own behavioral rehearsal will be correct. Also, seeing the wrong approach clearly displayed brings the ineffectiveness of it to the foreground.

Next, the couples themselves are instructed to take turns in the behavioral rehearsal of negative feelings. You will want to maintain a sense of reality in these practice sessions. A good rule of thumb is to have the couple replay situations that have actually occurred, either recently or recurrently in the past.

You may want to start by gaining some firsthand knowledge regarding the types of conflict that occur in the marriage. It usually does not pay to dwell on old wounds, to repeat hurts from past years that are no longer a living reality in the household. For purposes of therapy and attempts to enrich the relationship, it is much better to explore and deal with current frictions. You may ask each spouse what conflicts occurred during the past week and look for information about the problems that affect the couple in their daily relationship here and now.

Sometimes, current problems are easily dismissed by the couple as items of no real importance. However, often this dismissal is motivated by the fear of having yesterday's unpleasant scene recur in the therapist's office. And now without reason! The pain is fresh, the details are sharp in each one's mind, and not enough time has elapsed to allow the process of rationalization to safely throw all blame on the other. Practicing with "live ammunition" should not make the couple fearful but should remind you to proceed with caution.

The partners might benefit from a "dry run" in which they demonstrate how they did it incorrectly before trying to improve the performance. There is little need for contrived situations. Since the couple came for marital therapy, almost daily frictions are likely, and they should be dealt with in each session. Sometimes, a couple may feel so happy with the previously practiced exchange of positive feelings and the satisfactions gained from making positive requests that they are reluctant to embark on the risky journey of expressing negative feelings. However, the issues that cause tension have to be faced, and it is better to face them in the relative safety of your office under your careful guidance than at home, where long-lasting hurt is much more likely to occur.

When you start involving the marriage partners directly in behavioral rehearsal, it is a good idea to have one partner play the other partner's part, while you take the complementary role. This has the advantage of having each partner gain insight into how he or she is being perceived by the other and yet of avoiding a too-personal situation. As the therapist, you should take the part of the spouse who is trying to express negative feelings in the first rounds of practice. Of course, it is not wise to spend too much time with one partner or with one particular problem. The role playing can be kept profitably brief—less than 10 minutes for any particular interaction. Using a variety of problems that the couple is facing is creative and facilitates generalization beyond the therapy setting.

After some practice with you, the marriage partners will be able to role-play a situation together. Again, reversal of roles is often advisable at first. Because of the previous practice of positive exchanges, a reservoir of good feelings, your presence (and possibly that of other couples), and the structure of the procedure, there is little chance that the partners will antagonize each other. Usually, the spouses approach this phase of therapy with discretion and, at times, too much inhibition. Still, you should be cautious and intervene immediately when the role playing and practice degenerate into hostile feelings. If this should occur, the role play should be interrupted and the emotional situation briefly discussed without placing blame on either partner. A constructive approach for you to use at an inflammatory point such as this is to list a series of alternative ways in which the problem could have been handled. The "What if . . ." and "I also could have . . ." manner of looking at a conflict reduces anger and increases a rational outlook.

An additional warning for you as the therapist concerns our

professional tendency to escape into rationalization or excessive explanation and discussion. It is no doubt valid to explore the reasons that the spouses react the way they do, to understand the power lines of interaction, and to look carefully at the types of reactions that are elicited by given behaviors or expressions. However, it is all too easy to avoid the hard and serious work of practicing new behaviors to deal with old problems by talking about them or by talking about vaguely related matters. Your time and that of the couple are too valuable, and the problems facing the marriage too urgent, to permit any of you the luxury of lengthy armchair discussions. Insight will come quickly enough as the couple practice new and better ways of communicating.

It is important to remember that the clients may experience a variety of problems in connection with learning to express negative feelings. One or both partners may be afraid to deal with the problem; they may have to break long-established habits; they may lack awareness of their own negative feelings from lifelong suppression; and they may lack the appropriate social skills to work out a conflict-laden relationship. At all times, a careful and well-timed therapeutic approach is essential.

The recommended sequence (see Table V) for you to follow in directing the couple in behavioral rehearsal of negative feelings is:

1. The therapist models in a clear manner both appropriate and inappropriate ways of expressing negatives. It is a good idea to point out to the spouses what you will be demonstrating before modeling it and then afterwards to ask them what they observed.
2. The therapist and one client role-play. The therapist assumes

TABLE V. Checklist of Therapist Skills in Doing Active Behavioral Marital Therapy

________	1. Setting or eliciting goals for clients.
________	2. Offering or eliciting suggested scenes for clients to rehearse.
________	3. Structuring clients' role playing.
________	4. Instructing clients.
________	5. Modeling for the clients.
________	6. Prompting the clients.
________	7. Coaching or shadowing clients.
________	8. Giving clients positive feedback for specific behaviors.
________	9. Giving clients negative feedback for specific behaviors.
________	10. Behavioral rehearsals by clients.
________	11. Ignoring inconsequential or transient inappropriate behavior.
________	12. Getting physically within one foot of the clients during behavioral rehearsals.

the client's role and demonstrates the desired communication while the client takes his/her partner's role.

3. Same as (2) above, but now the client assumes his/her own position.
4. The two marriage partners role-play together with roles reversed.
5. Each partner takes his/her own role and practices a real situation that has occurred in the recent past.

An essential aspect of the communication of negative feelings is the feedback from the receiving partner. You should get the target of the negative emotions to tell the other how the experience made him/her feel. This process will help further to develop accurate empathy. Remember that empathy has two components:

1. The cognitive, which increases the receiving party's awareness of the sender's thoughts, opinions, and feelings.
2. The affective, which sensitizes the receiver to experiencing the actual feelings the sender has. When one spouse, under your guidance, learns how to verbalize negative feelings appropriately, the other can acquire both the cognitive and the affective elements of empathy much more easily.

— • —

Let's see an example of how a therapist might coach a couple in the constructive and assertive expression of negative feelings.

Husband: *I was really upset when you didn't want to answer the phone last night when I called. I knew you were home, so there was no reason.*
Wife: *You are too suspicious.*
Therapist: (To wife.) *Avoid accusations. Can you describe your feelings?*
Wife: *I feel as if you don't trust me. Yes, I was home, but I had fallen asleep with the TV on and I didn't hear the phone.*
Therapist: (To the husband.) *Can you give feedback?*
Husband: (Looking at therapist.) *She fell asleep in . . .*
Therapist: (Interrupting.) *Remember, look at your wife and tell her!*
Husband: *You were watching TV and did not hear the phone.*
Therapist: *What about her feelings?*
Husband: *But I do trust her!* (To his wife.) *I told you so over and over again. Just don't leave me hanging somewhere.*
Therapist: (Insisting.) *Tell your wife how you heard she felt.*

Husband: *You said that you feel as if I don't trust you.*
Therapist: *Good! Now, do you know what she means? If not, ask her.*
Husband: *What do you mean by not feeling trusted?*
Wife: *I feel that if I am not right there when you come home or call, you think I am running around town.*
Therapist: (To husband.) *Now, tell her how you feel about this.*
Husband: *I feel that I want to trust you, but you don't tell me anymore what you are doing and where you are going.*
Therapist: (To wife.) *Feedback, please.*
Wife: *You feel you want to trust me, but I don't tell you enough about what I'm doing.*
Therapist: (To wife.) *Do you feel you have enough personal freedom?*

From there followed an exploration of each partner's own rights and responsibilities and their shared time as a couple. Of special relevance were the issues presented in Chapter 3, "Planning Recreational and Leisure Time." The fact that the wife recently had been participating in assertiveness training groups for women had significant bearings on the case. She had become more aware of her own needs and growth possibilities, while he still thought of her in terms of the quiet, submissive homemaker he had married 15 years before. Appropriate expressions of negative feelings should not hurt or cause anger, while inappropriate expression is likely to incite anger, irritation, and a desire for counteraggression and retaliation.

———•———

During the behavior rehearsal, you, as the therapist, will prompt the clients, repeatedly model the correct behavior, and provide ample reinforcement when the appropriate behavior is approximated. If the spouses get into a rut, stop the action and model an alternative behavior, or have another client do the modeling if you are running a couples group. Then, return again to the person having the difficulty. Similarly, prompting and modeling may be necessary to obtain correct reactions from the spouse who is serving as the receiver or target of the anger. The receiving partner is to react by giving empathy, by reflecting back, by sharing meaning, or by checking out. For example, a good reaction would be "Did you mean that you felt bad when I spent an hour talking to that woman at the party?"

MARITAL THERAPY IN GROUPS

When other couples are receiving therapy at the same time, they should be involved in giving feedback (especially, positive feedback for approximations to improved expressions). You may prompt the other couples to share their own experiences and to model other ways of expressing negatives. To begin the learning process in a group, co-therapists may model a few conflict situations before asking the couples to rehearse their own problem scenes.

A particularly useful tool during the training of expression of negatives is audiotape or videotape feedback. The direct feedback, the accuracy of the recording, and the objectivity of the machine are very helpful in teaching clients to detect nonverbal elements of communication, such as tone of voice, interruptions, body posture, and gestures. Many people are a bit uncomfortable when hearing their own voices or seeing themselves on the monitor. Therefore, you may want to approach this technique in an easygoing, almost playful manner, and you should make sure that your voice and actions are recorded and played back several times before the clients are asked to participate. Audio and video recorders should not be used without clearly introducing the purposes you have in mind for them. The clients have to be able to trust their therapist, so they should know exactly when the recorder is used and what will happen with the recordings, especially after the therapy has terminated.

In terms of technique, you should get out of your seat often and actively work with your clients. The techniques of shadowing, prompting, and modeling are much more effective when you move from spouse to spouse and at times when you take the part of a spouse rather than simply give advice and interpretations. The methods used by the athletic or drama coach are a better model for the behavioral therapist than those of the film director or the psychoanalyst.

——— • ———

Let's see how an active therapist uses some of these methods:

Wife: *Our executive session did not go very well yesterday.*
Therapist: *Let's replay it here and see.*
Wife: *Okay.* (To husband in angry voice.) *You did not do any of the chores around the house this week and I feel as if you are taking me for granted.*
Therapist: (To wife.) *Let me take your place for a moment, and you watch how I avoid all accusations.*
Therapist: (Taking seat of wife.) *I really feel bad about something, Paul. Can we talk about that?*
Husband: (Nods.)
Therapist: (As wife.) *You know that I like to keep the house in good repair and I appreciate the help you usually*

give. But this week I missed your support and I felt neglected. (To wife.) *OK, now you do it.*

Wife: *I really feel bad about something . . .*

Therapist: (Moves over slightly behind and whispers.) *Look at him and turn more toward him. Good!*

Wife: (Continuing.) *You know that I like to keep the house clean and I missed your help this week.*

Therapist: (Prompting.) *Tell him that you like him to help you and how that makes you feel.*

Wife: *I really like it when we can do this together; it makes me feel real close to you—like taking care of the house is teamwork because the house is home for both of us.*

—— • ——

Look over the checklist of therapist skills in Table V and see how many you are doing now in your practice of marital therapy. How many do you have to learn?

THE ART OF REFRAMING

In any form of communication, perceptions of meaning—how the message is received and reacted to—is frequently dependent on the interpretation of the words and phrases by the listener. While the way in which the speaker uses verbal and nonverbal means to convey meaning is important, the filters and sensitivity and imputations of the listener often determine the impact of a message. The very same verbal content may be perceived very differently by people who are at different vantage points. Almost 2,000 years ago, Epictetus pointed out how spouses' personal perceptions of events and communication can interfere with a marriage when he wrote, "Men are disturbed not by things but by the views they take of them." From a therapeutic point of view, training spouses in marital communication should include helping them change the way they label their experiences. Watzlawick, Weakland, and Fisch (1974) presented the therapeutic value of "the gentle art of reframing" as enabling communicators to change their vantage points. They define *reframing* as changing a person's conceptual or emotional viewpoint or experience of a situation and placing it in another frame.

The process of reframing does not alter the facts of a situation, nor does it necessarily change any element in the situation; in fact, the situation may be unchangeable. The change effected by reframing is in the meaning attributed to the situation by the sender and the receiver of communications. An excerpt from Mark Twain's *The Adventures of Tom Sawyer* nicely illustrates the effectiveness of reframing:

It is Saturday afternoon, holiday time for all boys, except for Tom Sawyer, who has to whitewash 30 yards of board fence nine feet high. With this chore, life seems hollow, and existence a burden to Tom. It is not only the work that he finds intolerable but especially the thought of all the boys who will be coming along and making fun of him for having to work:

> At this dark and hopeless moment, an inspiration bursts upon him! Nothing less than a great, magnificent inspiration. Soon enough, a boy comes in sight, the very boy, of all boys, whose ridicule he had been dreading most.
>
> "Hello, old chap, you got to work, hey?"
>
> "Why, it's you, Ben! I warn't noticing."
>
> "Say,—I'm going a-swimming. *I* am. Don't you wish you could? But of course you'd druther *work*—wouldn't you? Course you would!"
>
> "Tom contemplated the boy a bit and said, "What do you call work?"
>
> "Why, ain't *that* work?"
>
> Tom resumed his whitewashing and answered carelessly, "Well, maybe it is, and maybe it ain't. All I know is, it suits Tom Sawyer."
>
> "Oh, come, now, you don't mean to let on that you *like* it?"
>
> The brush continued to move.
>
> "Like it? Well, I don't see why I oughtn't to like it. Does a boy get a chance to whitewash a fence every day?"
>
> *That put the thing in a new light.* Ben stopped nibbling his lunch while Tom swept his brush daintily back and forth—stepped back to note the effect—added a touch here and there—criticized the effect again—Ben watching every move and getting more and more interested, more and more absorbed.
>
> Presently he said, "Say, Tom, let *me* whitewash a little."

By the middle of the afternoon, the fence has three coats of whitewash and Tom is literally rolling in wealth, since one boy after another has parted with his riches for the privilege of painting a part of the fence. Tom succeeded in *reframing* drudgery as a pleasure for which one has to pay, and his friends have followed this change of his definition of reality.

Reframing is a procedure that intervenes at the cognitive level and gives the spouse permission to see a problem or some verbal message in a different light. The reinterpretation given by the therapist, like the one given by Tom Sawyer in the vignette quoted above, is usually more favorable and benign than the initial label used by the spouse. A well-known example of reframing a marital problem to a more benevolent situation is attributed to the creative therapist Milton Erickson (Johnson & Alevizos, 1975):

> A newly married man and his wife came to treatment because of the husband's impotence during their honeymoon. The husband had married his wife, who was a very beautiful young woman, after a long and sexually active and varied bachelorhood. The impotence was a great surprise to both the husband and his young wife; however, she felt insulted by his failure to perform sexually and was considering annulment. The husband was distraught by his sexual problem and at the prospect of losing his wife. Erickson saw each spouse separately and commented to both of them on what a great compliment the husband had paid to his wife in being so awestruck by her beauty that he was unable to do anything. That simple reinterpretation was immediately effective in reversing the husband's impotence.

By demonstrating the technique of reframing to your clients, you can help them understand that the way in which we label or view a given situation can determine the situation's impact on us. Few spouses will learn how to use the skill of reframing in their own marriage, since this requires a rather high level of sophistication on their part. We strongly recommend, however, that you, as the therapist, practice the art of reframing. When doing this, the rephrasing should not be seen by the spouses as a criticism of their expression, or a correction of their language skills, or as "a way in which you say things in the office," but as a way to understand a problem in a more agreeable and acceptable light.

One of us was once working with a client who stated in desperation, "I guess I was not meant to be happy in marriage!" Whereupon the therapist replied, "You mean that you want to get more out of the relationship than you are getting now?" A sudden surprise in the eyes of the unhappy spouse indicated the change that was brought about by reframing, by viewing the situation in a new light. Once a problem has been successfully reframed, it is often not so hard to think of ways to improve the situation.

Another opportunity for reframing comes when a spouse complains about how much of a struggle it is to follow through on homework assignments and how difficult it is to express feelings directly. You can reframe the complaint by stating, "I know it's a hard and a long haul, but people generally get more satisfaction in the end if they've first put out a lot of effort." One wife was complaining about how, at that point in therapy, she seemed to be making a disproportionate contribution to the initiation of positive communication while her husband was somewhat aloof. It was pointed out to her, in a separate individual visit, that this probably indicated that she had more power and strength for making changes than her husband at this time and could "afford" to carry a bigger share of the marital effort.

Reframing will be beneficial throughout the total process of marital therapy. Each therapist should be able to cite instances where helping a client adopt a different vantage point resulted in an improved disposition, mood, and outcome. If spouses can learn, through reframing, to change their perspective in their daily lives, many potential fights will be prevented. Mutual understanding—possibly with a bit of humor in addition—will be substituted for anger, boredom, or resentment.

SUMMARY

This chapter has emphasized the teaching of the expressive skills necessary for effective communication in marriage. Because these skills are not learned earlier in life by spouses in distressed marriages, they need to be systematically taught through instructions, modeling, coaching, feedback, and homework assignments.

The communication process is complex, and stages include expressing PLEASES, acknowledging PLEASES, asking for PLEASES, expressing negative feelings, empathy, sexual communication, and coping with unexpected hostility or persistent bad moods. Each of these types of communication can be taught through social learning principles and personal effectiveness techniques. The amount gained in therapy by any one spouse or couple will vary enormously, but each person should be able to make some degree of improvement in her or his communication skills. Starting with each client where he or she "is at," striving for small increments of change, and using a highly structured training program will bring increases in marital satisfaction for almost all couples. Whether the amount of improvement in satisfaction warrants the effort required to acquire and maintain it remains a question that each spouse must answer when therapy is terminated.

The nonverbal elements of communication—vocal volume and tone, eye contact, facial expressions, gestures, and body posture—are highlighted. Physical caressing and sex initiation exercises form a part of communication skills training in marriage therapy. A gradual approach to greater intimacy and mutual comfort is presented, with the therapist serving as a sensitive guide. Other sections suggest homework assignments and propose specific guidelines for marital therapy in groups.

The executive session, a structured interaction between the marriage partners, facilitates the learning of positive marital communication. The executive session has three components: receiving a message, processing it, and sending back a response. Topics and directions for executive sessions are suggested, and a homework report form is provided for spouses in the "Client's Workbook." After the couple(s) have acquired enough proficiency in communication to exchange negative feelings without provoking anger or resentment, the executive sessions may be omitted during therapy hours. However, it is usually best to request that the clients continue the sessions two or three times a week throughout the duration of therapy.

Of particular importance to successful marriages is the ability of spouses to express negative feelings. The marriage partners should realize that whenever strong negative emotions are aroused, the spouse experiencing the feeling can signal to the other the desire and need for an executive session. This does not mean that each time something negative comes up, a session has to be held. Most small and insignificant negative or hurt feelings can simply be ignored. It takes some discussion with the clients to help them discriminate important from insignificant negative feelings and occurrences. Even small negatives—for example, leaving socks out on the floor—can become significant and emotionally loaded if they occur frequently enough or if previous efforts to rectify them using straightforward, positive requests have failed. However, time *does* solve problems in many cases, and the spouses should realize that sometimes a little patience can go a long way. *Ignoring* temporary disturbing factors or *reframing* unpleasant events so that they are seen as small and insignificant will often obviate the need for protracted interactions or executive sessions.

The guidelines for effective communication that you, as the therapist, will emphasize in the course of marital treatment include the following:

1. It is better to make a request than a demand. A request shows respect for your spouse and encourages cooperation.
2. Ask questions; do not make accusations. Accusations only make your spouse defensive and rarely help in finding the "truth."
3. In talking about your partner's behavior, it is always more productive to speak of what he/she *does* rather than what he/she *is*. A label is rarely helpful in effecting behavior change.
4. Do not gunnysack; that is, don't bottle up resentments. In an argument, these bottled-up emotions are likely to be spilled out all at once, leading to destructive hostility.
5. During an argument, stick to the issue at hand; avoid piling one accusation on top of another.

6. Avoid excessive generalizations. Words such as *always* and *never* are often not true; besides, they frequently distract attention from the behavior and tend to label the person.
7. In every marital relationship, there should be "measured" honesty. Some things should never be said.

More time in marital therapy is devoted to training in communication skills because our clients have indicated that this is the most important part of their therapy experience. After considerable clinical efforts, we now feel that repeated practice and overlearning of communication skills will facilitate the durability and generality of improvements in marriage relationships.

REFERENCES

GENERAL

Johnson, S. M., & Alevizos, P. N. *Strategic therapy: A systematic outline of procedures.* Paper presented at the Ninth Annual Conference of the Association for the Advancement of Behavior Therapy, San Francisco, December 1975.

Miller, S., Nunnally, E. W., & Wackman, D. B. *Alive and aware: Improving communication in relationships.* Minneapolis: Interpersonal Communication Programs, Inc., 1975.

Rogers, C., & Stevens, B. *Person to person: The problem of being human.* Lafayette, Calif.: Real People Press, 1967.

Watzlawick, P., Weakland, J., & Fisch, R. *Change: Principles of problem formation and problem resolution.* New York: Norton, 1974.

SEX THERAPY

Annon, J. *Behavioral treatment of sexual problems: Brief therapy.* New York: Harper & Row, 1976.

Caird, W., & Wincze, J. P. *Sex therapy: A behavioral approach.* New York: Harper & Row, 1977.

Fischer, R., & Gochros, G. *A handbook of behavior therapy with sexual problems.* New York: Pergamon, 1978.

Heiman, J., LoPiccolo, L., & LoPiccolo, J. *Becoming orgasmic: A sexual growth program for women.* Englewood Cliffs, N.J.: Prentice-Hall, 1976.

Kaplan, H. S. *The new sex therapies.* New York: Brunner/Mazel, 1974.

Kaplan, H. S. *The illustrated manual of sex therapy.* New York: Quadrangle/New York Times Book Co., 1975.

Kass, D. J., & Stauss, F. F. *Sex therapy at home.* New York: Simon & Schuster, 1975.

McCarthy, B. W., Ryan, M., & Johnson, F. A. *Sexual awareness—A practical approach.* San Francisco: Boyd and Fraser, 1975.

NEGATIVE FEELINGS

Bach, G. R. & Goldberg, H. *Creative aggression*. New York: Avon, 1974.

Bach, G. R., & Wyden, P. *The intimate enemy: How to fight fair in love and marriage*. New York: Avon, 1968.

Human Development Institute. *Improving communication in marriage*. Atlanta, 1967.

Stuart, R. B., & Lederer, G. *How to make a bad marriage good and a good marriage better*. New York: Putnam, 1978.

Viscott, D. *How to live with another person*. New York: Arbor House and Pocket Books, 1974, 1976.

CHAPTER 6

Giving and Getting: Marital Contracts

The contracting process can be one of the most important skills that couples learn in therapy. Contracts between marriage partners are not a new or revolutionary idea. The *ketubah*, the ancient Jewish marriage contract, determined certain obligations of husband and wife to one another. As tribes and clans evolved into political entities, the state began to dictate how individuals were to become and remain married. In this way, many provisions from ancient marriage contracts were assimilated into legal statutes or common law, while others continued as traditions or customs. Thus, the revival of personal contracts between marriage partners has historical precedent. One difference between the historical and current therapeutic use of marriage contracts is that contemporary contracting is done with couples who are already married and who are experiencing discomfort in their relationship.

Contracting between spouses in marital therapy can be a simple and expedient way to harness the natural rewards present in the marital relationship. Contracts structure interpersonal exchanges between partners in terms of *who* does *what* to *whom* and *when*. Behaviors or actions and their positive consequences are clearly delineated. The end product of contracting is a written agreement for behavior change by both partners that is understandable and acceptable to each spouse. At the end of the contracting process, each partner will have a separate contract specifying at least two privileges that are contingent on carrying out two corresponding responsibilities. However, a contract as an *end product* is not nearly as valuable as practicing and learning the skills of specification, negotiation, and compromise that occur during the *process* of contracting.

Contracting as it is used here has two goals. First and foremost, the contracting process opens up communication between partners experiencing difficulties in their relationship. Under the guidance of the therapist, each spouse requests in nonthreatening, positive ways, certain actions by the other that will begin to make their relationship more rewarding. Spouses begin to specify, perhaps for the first time, what they want from each other as well as what they are really willing to give to each other. Second, the process is structured to teach couples how to use contracting as a problem-solving tool to deal with differences when they arise. In this way, it becomes a process for managing conflict in the present and in the future. Negotiation, bargaining, empathizing, and compromising are modeled and reinforced by the therapist during the contracting process. The ultimate effectiveness of the contracting process is directly related to the extent to which these interpersonal skills generalize to problem solving and conflict management in the home.

To meet these goals, the contracting process is broken down into a series of counseling sessions. In early sessions, spouses negotiate and make agreements under the direct supervision of the therapist for mutual exchanges of responsibilities and privileges that are likely to cause little disagreement and in which the spouses have little emotional investment. In later sessions, the emotional loading of topics is increased, while the negotiation still takes place under the supervision of the therapist. After succeeding at this level, the couple are encouraged to use the contracting process at home as issues arise and to report back on their progress at counseling sessions. This sequencing is very important for several reasons: for example, preventing failure, encouraging continuation of practice, rewarding success, and strengthening recent learning.

The therapist is teaching a husband and wife a new skill. Therefore, the contracting process needs to be broken down into small, manageable steps to increase the probability that the couple will experience early success with it. Success makes the process rewarding for the couple and increases their motivation to use it when the issues to be negotiated are more emotionally charged and difficult to arrange. As a byproduct of initial successes, the couple perceive their relationship becoming more viable and positive as each gives and gets more.

MAKING POSITIVE REQUESTS

The first step in initiating couples into the contracting procedure is to help them make *positive* requests of each other. The executive session format, covered in Chapter 5, is used at this stage. To demonstrate that they are developing adequate listening and reflecting skills, a couple need to practice making positive requests during executive sessions at home for at least one week. In instructing the couple to make requests of each other, you might emphasize that requests are more effective when they are worded positively. In other words, each spouse is urged to say what is wanted from the partner rather than what is not wanted. Asking a spouse to stop doing something elicits a defense of these actions rather than a willingness to consider changing in the future. For example, when Arthur asked Mary to "stop being so sloppy around the house," her response was to begin defending herself and attacking him for not picking up his clothes, shoes, and correspondence. However, when Arthur was able to reword the request to "I would really appreciate it if you would pick up the living room before I get home at night," Mary was more receptive and able to consider the request.

Requests should be made in terms of specific behaviors rather than general personality characteristics. Asking a husband to be "more considerate" is too vague for him to understand what his wife wants him to *do* differently and may make him feel attacked. The vague phrase "more considerate" may mean anything from "put your dirty clothes in the hamper" to "come home from work on time" to "listen to me talk about my day for a few minutes." It is up to you, as the therapist, to help the wife in this situation to specify what *actions* she wants her husband to engage in, *how often*, *when*, and *where*, that will make him appear "more considerate."

Positive requests should be limited to one week. There is more chance for practice and for success if the behaviors requested are likely to occur several times in the coming week.

To further illustrate these instructions, you, as the therapist, may demonstrate an inappropriate and an appropriate way of making such a request. For example, how *not* to do it!

THERAPIST: *(Modeling for wife.)* It was so unusual for you to come home from work on time yesterday that I almost couldn't believe my eyes. From now on, I would like you to stop being inconsiderate and to stop coming home late so often.

This request is worded negatively rather than positively. It does not specify the behavior to be increased or decreased but, instead, asks for a change in motivation (inconsiderateness) and is not time-limited. This type of request is likely to initiate defensiveness rather than compliance on the part of the partner at whom it is aimed.

Now you may demonstrate how the same request could be made to increase the likelihood that the person hearing the request will agree or be willing to negotiate: How to *do* it!

THERAPIST: *(Modeling for wife.)* I really liked your coming home on time yesterday. I would like you to come home on time or call if you are going to be more than half an hour late any night for the next week. This would make my evenings start more happily.

This request is worded positively. It specifies the behaviors to be increased and is time-limited. It opens the way for the partner to respond in several ways. First, using the executive session format, he must reflect back or paraphrase the request. Then, he may agree to do it four out of five nights for the next week and request a privilege in exchange. For example, he may request that his spouse greet him with a hug and a smile on those days he comes home on time or calls her. He can explain that a warm greeting makes his evening start more happily and makes him feel good. He now has the first term in a contract. His responsibility of coming home on time is specified, and he has chosen a specific privilege that he would like in return.

Once you have explained and demonstrated the procedure, have the couple try this in the session with you, coaching both partners as they make their requests and reflect back their partner's requests. Each partner should have a chance to make one request during the session for the coming week without necessarily tying it together with a privilege!

—— • ——

The following dialogue is between Arthur and Mary Peabody when they tried this procedure for the first time under the therapist's supervision:

Therapist: Now that we've talked about and demonstrated how to use your executive sessions to make requests of each other, I'd like you to try it. You begin, Mary. Begin with a statement of positive feelings and then make a request. Arthur will reflect back to you what he heard you say before responding to your request.

Mary: *It would make me feel good if you wouldn't turn away and read the paper or walk off when I try and tell you about my day at home with the kids.*

Therapist: *Mary, you told him what you didn't want. What do you want him to do instead? Start again.*

Mary: *It would make me feel important if you would listen to me once in a while when I try to tell you about my day.*

Therapist: Better.

Arthur: *I hear you say that you would like me to listen to you when you want to tell me about your day.*

Therapist: *Is that what you said, Mary?*

Mary: Yes.

Therapist: *Now, it's your turn, Arthur. State how that makes you feel.*

Arthur: *I find it really upsetting to be greeted at the door with a long list of complaints about your day. I'm tired when I come home and need a few minutes to unwind.*

Mary: *Well, I'm tired, too, and* . . . (Interrupted by therapist.)

Therapist: *Mary, reflect back when you heard him say.*

Mary: *I heard you say that you don't like to listen to me complain when you first come home because you're tired and need some time to yourself.*

Therapist: *That's good, Mary. Now, state your request in more specific terms. How often, when, and for how long would you like Arthur to listen to you talk about your day?*

Mary: *I would like you to listen to me for about ten minutes every day. I understand that you're tired when you come home, so maybe we could make it after dinner.*

Therapist: *Add how that would make you feel, why it's important.*

Mary: *It would make me feel as if I matter and as if what goes on at home is important to you.*

Therapist: Good.

Arthur: *I hear you say that you would like me to listen to you for ten minutes every evening after dinner and that would make you feel as if you matter.*

Therapist: *Very good. Now, Arthur, you may respond to the request by agreeing or making a counterproposal for more or less time or more or less often. You may also make a request for something in return—you mentioned something about time to unwind when you get home.*

Arthur: *I can understand how that would make you feel as if I'm interested in you. I can go along with that to see how it works for a week. I come home from work very uptight, and I would like to have fifteen minutes every day when I first come home to be left alone by the kids and everyone to unwind. I think that would put me in a better mood for the evening.*

Mary: *I hear you say that you would be willing to try this arrangement for a week and that you would like fifteen minutes of uninterrupted time to unwind when you come home every day. I'll agree to that.*

Therapist: *It sounds as if you have come to an agreement that you are both willing to try for one week. You will both be giving something and getting something. Report back next week on how it went.*

Below are some examples of the requests that couples have made of each other:

Wife of husband

1. "I would appreciate your picking up your dishes and putting them in the sink after dinner."
2. "I would like you to compliment me on my appearance once a day."
3. "I would like it if you would kiss me good-bye in the morning."
4. "I would like you to get the kids ready for bed two evenings next week."
5. "I would like you to get up with the baby and let me sleep in on Sunday morning."

Husband of wife

1. "I would like you to cook spaghetti for dinner once a week; it's my favorite meal."
2. "I would like you to sit and watch the news with me after dinner."
3. "I would like you to plan an evening out this week, just the two of us."
4. "I would like you to make a big breakfast on Sunday morning."
5. "I would like a ten-minute back rub twice a week in the evening."

GUIDELINES FOR CONTRACTING IN MARITAL GROUPS

1. Begin the request procedure with a couple who are likely to respond well to your instructions and prompts. That is, start with a couple who will be a good model for other group members.
2. Have each couple make their requests in turn as you proceed around the group. Ask other group members to give feedback to the couple spotlighted regarding the specificity of the request being made. Cut off value judgments by group members as to the appropriateness of the request.
3. When the request is made and agreed upon by both parties, encourage supportive remarks by other group members.

THE CONTRACTING EXERCISE

During this phase, the couple will be engaging in a formal contracting exercise that culminates in a written contract specifying responsibilities, privileges, bonuses, and negative consequences for each partner.

The first step is to introduce the idea of contracting to the couple. There are four basic guidelines for effective contracts (DeRisi & Butz, 1975; Homme, 1969; Stuart, 1971). First, the negotiation must be open, honest, and free from explicit or subtle coercion. For example, a husband may be subtly coerced to ask his wife to "initiate sex twice a week," not because he really cares but because the popular press tells him this is how sex *should* be between husband and wife. Each spouse must be honest about what he or she wants and is willing to give if the contract is to be realistic. Second, the terms of the contract should be written simply, explicitly, and clearly. No fine print! Vague, general terms lead to misunderstandings later when spouses try to decide if they have fulfilled their end of the agreement. For example, a contract in which a husband agrees to "pay more attention to the kids" is destined to failure, since his idea of "more attention" may differ greatly from his wife's definition of the term. The terms should be explicit, such as "husband agrees to play a game with children for 20 minutes each day," so that both parties understand clearly what they are agreeing to. Third, the contract must provide advantages to each spouse over the status quo. Each must feel that she or he has gained something of value in the relationship. This may be simply an increase in the frequency of an action that already occurs occasionally. For example, a wife may ask her husband to plan a leisure-time activity for the family every week instead of once a month, which he currently does. Fourth, the behavior contracted must be in the current repertoire of the person agreeing to it. For example, don't ask an impotent husband to initiate and carry out sex twice a week.

To set favorable expectations, you should clarify the value of contracting to the couple and point out how it serves several purposes. The contracting process teaches spouses *specificity* in asking for what each partner needs from the other. It also teaches the important *negotiation skills* of communicating desires directly, nonaccusatorily and of giving positive and negative feedback to a spouse during negotiations. Contracting also gives the couple experience in *agreeing* on those issues that initially sparked differences. A good contract represents a successful compromise where both spouses feel they get something by giving something.

These skills are the essence of successful communication and problem solving in marriage. The contracting procedure is aimed at starting or accelerating these skills so that later, after practice, experience, and success, this process can be done effectively by the spouses themselves in a more spontaneous, less directive manner. You should stress that couples who succeed at negotiating a successful contract during the workshop have the best prognosis for improving their marriage. Thus, contracting serves a diagnostic and prognostic function as well as a therapeutic function.

Once the rationale for contracting is explained and understood by the couple, focus the couple's attention on the "Family Happiness Index" (see Table VI). The "Family Happiness Index" has examples of many types of requests that partners in a marriage may want to make of each other. A copy of the "Family Happiness Index" is included in the "Client's Workbook."

Using the "Family Happiness Index" during these initial steps in teaching contracting has several advantages. First, it provides a "menu" of possible behaviors that spouses may ask for or provide to each other and thus facilitates their thinking of something. Second, the items on the index are listed as discrete behaviors, reducing the chance that couples will launch into complex, multiple, or global requests, such as "I want you to be a better wife/husband." Since the Index is broken down into categories, it is diagnostic of the areas in which the couple is experiencing most difficulty as opposed to those areas where they are experiencing satisfaction.

TABLE VI. Family Happiness Index

Leisure-Time Management

1. Goes for a ride with me.
2. Gives me time alone.
3. Goes out to dinner with me.
4. Spends a weekend with me away from home.
5. Talks to me on the phone.
6. Goes out with me for entertainment.
7. Gives me time to be with my own friends alone.
8. Gives me time to work on my own hobby.
9. Plays sports with me.
10. Watches TV with me.

Household Chores

1. Does an errand.
2. Completes household repairs.
3. Cleans house better.

Auto and Transportation

1. Washes the car.
2. Gets the car fixed and serviced.
3. Meets me on time.
4. Gives me transportation money.

Sex and Affection

1. Initiates sexual advances.
2. Pleasantly responds to my advances.
3. Hugs and kisses me.
4. Surprises me with a gift.
5. Tells me I am loved.
6. Holds my hand.

Meals and Shopping

1. Shops with me.
2. Gets up and makes me breakfast.
3. Has dinner ready on time.
4. Cooks or bakes with me.

Personal Habits and Acceptance

1. Compliments my appearance.
2. Decreases drinking or smoking.
3. Wears pleasing attire.
4. Changes hairstyle.

Consideration and Attention

1. Converses with me.
2. Comes to bed with me.
3. Asks about my feelings.
4. Holds the door for me.

Care of Children

1. Plays with the children.
2. Disciplines the children with me.
3. Takes the children out or baby-sits.

Money Management

1. Plans the budget.
2. Takes responsibility for the checkbook and bills.
3. Gives me money to spend on a special treat.

After the couple have had a few moments to look over the "Family Happiness Index," explain the steps of the contracting procedure to be used over the next few sessions:

1. One spouse chooses one, two, or three behaviors or events from the Index that he/she "might" be willing to do and that he/she thinks would please the other spouse. These are potential "Responsibilities" in the final contract.
2. For these potential "Responsibilities," each spouse gets feed-

TABLE VII. *Schematic Outline of Contracting Exercise*

Husband		*Wife*
What does she want that I can offer?	Identifying responsibility for self.	What does he want that I can offer?
What do I want that she might do?	Identifying responsibility for spouse.	What do I want that he might do?
How much would I like her carrying out her responsibilities?	Setting values on responsibilities.	How much would I like his carrying out his responsibilities?
How hard would it be for me to carry mine out?	Setting costs on responsibilities.	How hard would it be for me to carry mine out?
How does she feel about her potential responsibilities?	Empathizing.	How does he feel about his potential responsibilities?
What would I want as a privilege or treat?	Identifying reward for self.	What would I want as a privilege or treat?
What would she want as a privilege or treat?	Identifying reward for spouse.	What would he want as a privilege or treat?
Which responsibility will be most difficult for me to implement?	Setting priorities on responsibilities.	Which responsibility will be most difficult for me to implement?
Which privilege do I want the most?	Setting priorities on privileges.	What privilege do I want the most?
What am I willing to give for what I want?	Bargaining and negotiating.	What am I willing to give for what I want?
Are the terms of the contract fair and balanced?	Compromising.	Are the terms of the contract fair and balanced?
Can I commit myself to the contract?	Agreement.	Can I commit myself to the contract?

back from his/her partner on how pleasing each event or behavior would be *if* it were done.

3. Each spouse chooses one, two, or three behaviors or events from the Index that would please himself or herself. These are potential "Privileges" in the final contract.
4. The partners put themselves in each other's place and describe why and how these potential privileges would please the other.
5. Each spouse explains how difficult it would be to carry out the chosen responsibilities.
6. Each spouse ranks the privileges as to their degree of desirability and the responsibilities as to their degree of difficulty.
7. Each spouse negotiates, compromises, and specifies the dimensions of how often, how much, when, where, and with whom.
8. Each spouse agrees to comply with the terms of the contract and to keep records on the performance of him/herself and spouse.

The entire contracting exercise is outlined in Table VII.

GUIDELINES FOR A GROUP FORMAT

When using the contracting exercise in a group workshop for couples, you may wish to use a large "Family Happiness Board" that can be seen by the entire group. The board, an enlarged representation of the "Family Happiness Index," is approximately 3′ × 5′ and can be hung on a wall or placed on an easel. Each of the affectional and behavioral categories is a potential request printed in large letters. Beside each item on the board is an envelope containing several 3″ × 5″ cards. The request is typed on the card along with blanks for the spouse to fill in with the specifics of how often, when, where, and with whom.

> ______________ converses with me
> how often? ______________
> when? ______________
> where? ______________

Using the board in a group allows all group members to see it at once, and the activity of each participant walking up and choosing a card provides an opportunity for mutual support and group discussion.

CHOOSING RESPONSIBILITIES

To start the couple in the contracting exercise, you pass out blank contracts with columns titled "Privileges" and "Responsibilities" (see the sample of blank contracts in the "Client's Workbook"). Let's now follow Arthur and Mary through the contracting process. We began by asking Mary and Arthur to each pick one behavioral item from the "Family Happiness Index" representing an action that each "might" carry out as a responsibility and that each thought would please the other. We cautioned them that the action chosen need not be a surprise or a fantastic gift but only something that might please the other. It is important to indicate that these are only *potential responsibilities,* being chosen in a preliminary phase of developing terms for a contract and that this initial choice does not bind them to comply with the responsibility until the exchange and negotiation process is completed.

We then asked Mary to read her chosen responsibility and to explain why she thought it would please Arthur. Mary picked "Initiates sex." The therapist then prompted Mary to make this potential action more specific, that is, to spell it out in terms of how often, when, and where. Mary offered to initiate sex once a week in the evening instead of about once a month, as she had been doing up to that time.

We then asked Arthur, who would be the beneficiary of Mary's potential increase in initiating sex, to give feedback on whether or not this would actually please him and to state how it would make him feel to receive it. Arthur said that Mary's initiating sex once a week would please him as it would make him feel attractive and desirable to her.

If the responsibility selected is not viewed as pleasing or desirable by the other spouse, then another one is selected and the above steps are repeated. This checking-out process keeps the marital exchanges on target and elucidates the needs, desires, priorities, and values of each partner, which, in the past, may have been covert, implicit, and misinterpreted. Since Arthur responded favorably to Mary's choice, she was asked to write the behavior under "Responsibilities" on her blank contract.

Arthur then read the potential responsibility he selected as possibly pleasing for Mary. Arthur selected "Takes children out or baby-sits." He specified that he would baby-sit or take their daughter out for one hour on a weekday evening and for two hours on the weekend. Mary accepted this offer, indicating that it would give her some free time to do things that she enjoys alone and that it would make her feel less hassled.

At the end of this stage, each spouse should have one specifically described behavior under the "Responsibilities" column of the contract form:

Arthur Peabody		*Mary Peabody*	
Responsibilities	Privileges	Responsibilities	Privileges
Takes child out or baby-sits one hour during week and two hours during weekend.		Initiates sex once a week in the evening.	

We then asked Arthur and Mary each to choose another behavior from the Index that described an action by their partner that would please them. That is, Mary chose an action that she would like Arthur to perform, and Arthur chose an action that he would like Mary to perform. This behavior should not be the same as a behavior chosen in the first step of the exercise. The spouses then take turns reading the behavior they would like to receive from the other and explaining why it is important. Arthur chose the behavior "Has dinner ready on time every evening" as something he would like Mary to do. He said that it was important to him because it makes him feel as though he matters to her, and, besides, he's hungry when he gets home at night. Mary chose "Compliments me on my appearance at least once a day" because that makes her feel desirable. These behavioral items were then exchanged, and Mary and Arthur put them in the "Responsibilities" column of their contracts. Make sure that all chosen responsibilities are realistic and possible. Reality-testing should be done on the action chosen as well as on the dimensions of how often, how much, when, where, and with whom. As the therapist, you want couples to experience some success in carrying out the contract, so they should be cautioned to scale it down if they are unsure of whether or not they can carry out an action. At this point, Arthur and Mary's potential contracts look like this:

Arthur Peabody		*Mary Peabody*	
Responsibilities	Privileges	Responsibilities	Privileges
1. Takes child out or baby-sits one hour during week and two hours during weekend.		1. Initiates sex once a week in the evening.	
2. Compliments Mary's appearance once a day.		2. Has dinner ready on time every night.	

The spouses now have two responsibilities on their respective contracts. The next step in the contracting exercise is designed to build empathy. Empathy is aided by having the partners publicly set costs or degrees of difficulty in carrying out the actions listed as responsibilities on each of the contracts.

To further this exchange of empathy, the contracts should be exchanged temporarily by the partners. Ask the spouses, in turn, to state how they would feel if their partner actually carried out the behaviors or actions described in the "Responsibilities" column of their respective contracts. Ask each partner to put herself or himself in the other's shoes and state how hard it would be for the other to carry out the potential responsibility. After each spouse has had an opportunity to do this, ask them to return the contracts to each other. Make sure that each spouse agrees that it would be possible and reasonable to carry out the two responsibilities listed on the contracts. Note that in the next phase of the contracting exercise, each would be getting something in return as a privilege. If agreement is obtained on the reasonableness of the stated responsibilities, have each spouse rank them according to the degree of difficulty anticipated in carrying them out. The more difficult responsibility is placed at the top of the column.

Arthur agreed that the responsibilities on his contract were reasonable, and he put them in the following order of difficulty:

1. Takes child out or baby-sits one hour during the week and two hours during the weekend
2. Compliments Mary on her appearance once a day

Mary felt that she might not be able to have dinner ready on time every night but could five nights out of seven. Arthur agreed to this, since it was an improvement over what she was currently doing. Mary ranked her responsibilities as:

1. Have dinner ready on time five nights out of seven
2. Initiate sex once a week

The contracts were put away until the next session, when the exercise would be completed by the selection of privileges and negotiating the agreement.

In the next session, return the contract forms to each spouse and have them review their stated responsibilities. Ask how they now feel about the two responsibilities listed and if their feelings have changed as a result of a week's thinking or interacting. If one spouse's feelings have changed, give her or him the opportunity to change the specifics of *how often, when,* and *where* or to choose another responsibility if the action is now viewed as inappropriate. If changes are made, provide guidance through the same process with the new "Responsibility." Once the responsibilities have been accepted, the couple is ready for the next step of choosing privileges.

CHOOSING PRIVILEGES

Before beginning the next step, remind the couple that the purpose of the exercise is to promote negotiation and compromise skills. The actual contract itself is of minimal value unless the couple learn in the process to specify and operationalize what they want from and are willing to give to each other. Make sure the couple learns to set realistic goals for responsibilities and privileges.

When this has been made clear, ask each spouse to pick a behavior from the "Family Happiness Index" representing an action that would be pleasing to herself or himself. This may be an action performed by herself or himself, some behavior performed by the other spouse, or some solitary or mutual activity. The privilege chosen may be an activity or a behavior that is currently being received or engaged in, but that the chooser desires to continue or to increase in frequency. Each spouse should be encouraged to ask, "What do I really want enough to work for?" A spouse may choose a novel behavior or activity if none of the existing items from the Index is appropriate. Remind each spouse to fill in the specifics of where, when, how often, and with whom for the chosen privilege. If necessary, coach the spouses to help them achieve specificity.

Each spouse now reads the privilege to the other and states why it is valued. Prompt the partners to ask themselves if the privilege requested is realistic and reasonable. You may need to assist the spouses in modifying the specifics so that their privileges can be made realistic. Mary chose "Going out to dinner once a week" as a privilege she would enjoy and be willing to work for. Arthur immediately brought up the budget. After some discussion, both agreed that they could afford to go out to dinner once a week at an inexpensive, family-type restaurant. This was still acceptable to Mary, since her main concern was not having to cook dinner. Arthur chose "Watches a sports event on TV with me once a week" as a privilege he would like Mary to provide for him, since he likes company while he watches TV and hopes she'll get more interested in sports.

If the chosen privilege is unrealistic and cannot be modified adequately, another privilege should be chosen. Praise the spouses for their honesty and openness, since the success of the contract depends on each party's being forthright about what is realistic for them at this time. An example of confronting an unrealistic contract was a wife who wanted the privilege of going to her mother's house two hours every day, even though she usually came home upset from these visits. Her husband at first rejected the request, but with the therapist's help, the privilege was modified to less frequent visits (once a week) but for a longer duration (five hours). When a behavior or activity is mutually acceptable, it is placed in the person's contract in the "Privileges" column.

The next step is for each spouse to pick a behavior from the Index that is likely to please the other. The specifics are filled in according to where, when, how often, how long, and with whom. The choosing spouse then reads the behavior aloud as a potential privilege for the other. The recipient may accept it; modify it according to frequency, setting, or intensity; or reject it and request that something else be substituted. If the privilege offered is accepted, have the receiving spouse state how this activity or behavior would please him/her. The recipient then takes the card and places it in his/her "Privileges" column.

Arthur chose "Money to spend on a special treat" as a potential privilege for Mary. More specifically, Mary wanted to go out to lunch with her girlfriends once a week without being hassled about the expense, and Arthur chose this as a privilege for Mary. Mary chose "Washes the car every week" as a privilege she would be willing to provide for Arthur, since "he hates to wash the car."

Make sure that each spouse agrees that it would be realistically possible to carry out the two listed privileges. Each spouse then ranks the two according to the amount of pleasure and reward that each would provide and places the more desirable privilege at the top of the column.

Mary ranked her privileges as:

1. Going out to dinner once a week
2. Money for a special treat

Arthur ranked his privileges as:

1. Watches a sports event on TV with me once a week
2. Mary washes the car

NEGOTIATING THE CONTRACT

The final step in the process is negotiating, bargaining, compromising, and, hopefully, agreeing. This is a critical step and deserves your close supervision. As the therapist, you may model this final phase to help ensure that spouses exchange feelings and ideas in ways that are consistent with the adaptive communication patterns already practiced in previous sessions (see Chapter 5). You may also need to coach one or both spouses earlier during the exchange of responsibilities and privileges to facilitate optimum communication. Further, the *contingencies* of the exchange process must be clearly spelled out. Each spouse must understand that:

1. Each partner must fulfill a responsibility before partaking of the attached privilege. Nothing comes free of charge. Each person earns a privilege by first carrying out the attendant responsibility.
2. Each partner must agree on how much of the responsibility earns how much of the privilege. For example, how many times does Sylvester have to take his wife out to dinner to earn a weekend of fishing alone with his friends? The contract cannot be actualized until both spouses understand and agree to the contingencies of the exchange process.

The contracting exercise is structured, but it requires flexibility to attain full agreement and commitment to the terms of the contract. Thus, couples should be allowed to substitute different privileges or responsibilities if the need arises. A bonus privilege may also be added as an extra incentive for a partner's compliance with the terms of his or her contract over several weeks. For example, if Mary has dinner ready six evenings a week for two weeks, Arthur might offer to take her to dinner at a fancy restaurant and a movie. If the couple is willing, a medium of exchange may be used to help them monitor their contract and gauge their daily progress. For example, every day that Mary has dinner ready on time, Arthur may give her a receipt. She keeps the receipts, and when she has collected the agreed-upon number of receipts, she can turn them in for her privilege of going out to dinner.

Mary would give Arthur a receipt every time he compliments her appearance, and when the specified number of receipts have been collected by Arthur, Mary will wash the car. For some couples, this medium of exchange feels too stilted. Do not force or push the idea of receipts on unwilling couples. For other couples, the idea of exchanging receipts or play money strikes them as fun and provides an easy way for them to monitor their progress on the contract.

The couple should be informed that they are expected to comply with the terms of the final contract for one week. For this reason, it is important that the privileges and responsibilities that are chosen occur at least once a week so that the contract can be tested out by the next session. At the next session, there will be an opportunity to renegotiate the contract terms.

Caution: It is important that the contract be parallel. This means that one person's responsibility cannot be the other's privilege. For example, Carla may have chosen cooking a special meal for her husband once a week as a responsibility. Thus, having a special meal prepared for him cannot be one of her husband's privileges, since he should not get that meal without first completing his corresponding responsibility. Parallel contracts allow each spouse to comply with the terms of his/her contract relatively independently and avoid recriminations over who did what first. While a husband may fail to comply with the terms of his contract, his wife could still comply with hers.

While the couple is negotiating the contract, the therapist should prompt and praise efforts at good verbal communication. Good verbal communication includes being specific, owning up to feelings, making requests directly, and giving and acknowledging PLEASES. When the negotiations are completed, the therapist may have the contracts typed up by a secretary while the session continues with other activities. When typed, the copies are signed, and each spouse takes one copy of each contract. Typing is certainly not essential, but the contracts should be written out for future reference and copies reserved for each spouse and the therapist.

As you review a completed contract, consider whether it contains the ingredients of a successful agreement:

1. Are the behavioral terms realistic and specific?
2. Are the responsibilities balanced by the privileges?
3. Is each privilege set up to be conditional on first completing the matching responsibility?
4. Does each spouse know how to monitor progress and compliance and report them to the therapist?
5. Have both partners practiced and learned the critical commu-

nication skills that are needed to deal constructively with conflict and to maintain positive reciprocity?

At the end of the exercise, Arthur's and Mary's contracts looked like this:

Mary Peabody

Responsibilities	Privileges
1. Have dinner ready by 6:00 P.M., five evenings of the week.	1. Go out to dinner to a moderately priced restaurant of her choice once a week.
2. Initiate sex once a week in the evening (not during a favorite TV program of Arthur's).	2. Money for lunch with her friends once a week (Arthur will not hassle her, but will say, "Have a good time").

Bonus: If Mary has dinner ready on time six evenings of the week for two weeks, Arthur will take her to dinner and a movie.

Arthur Peabody

Responsibilities	Privileges
1. Baby-sits one hour during the week and two hours during the weekend.	1. Mary watches two hours of a sporting event on TV with Arthur once a week (Monday night football) and makes popcorn.
2. Compliments Mary on her appearance (or some other *personal* compliment) once a day.	2. Mary washes the car once a week.

Bonus: If Arthur baby-sits an extra hour during the week, Mary will fix a "favorite meal" for him one night of the week.

Signed:

______________	______________	______
Mary Peabody	Arthur Peabody	Witness

Record sheets are provided for the couple to serve as checklists for compliance with the terms of the contract. Sample record sheets are provided in the "Client's Workbook." These sheets should be used daily at home as a reminder to follow through on the agreement made in the therapy session. The couple are encouraged to bring their record sheets to succeeding sessions as a way of reporting on their progress.

The advantages of conscientious and systematic monitoring of contracts are enumerated below. Record keeping facilitates adherence to contracts by:

1. Bridging the gap between treatment sessions and providing frequent feedback and visual evidence of progress throughout the week at the very times that the responsibilities and privileges are carried out.

2. Serving as a cue or reminder for the therapist and the couple to offer social reinforcement to each other. This cueing function generates chains of positive interactions that can help move the couple into new ways of relating.
3. Prompting new, more positive ways of relating that may replace coercive ways.
4. Prompting self-monitoring and self-reinforcement, which may lead to more durable changes at the end of therapy.
5. Providing feedback of progress to the therapist and extending the therapist's surveillance to cover more of the couple's interaction than just what is seen at the session.
6. Symbolically extending the presence of the therapist from the office into the natural milieu—especially if the record form is specially designed for the couple and if the therapist prompts between sessions by phone or mail.
7. Helping partners save face. Neither has to accept the blame for past problems. Neither has to take the sole responsibility for change. Neither is the designated patient. Marital partners can say, "We're doing it because it's in the contract and we both agreed to it."
8. Helping to keep the partners honest. There is a marked tendency to cheat, ignore, or forget the contract terms, even right after the agreement has been made. The influence of old behavior is great, and procrastination and vagueness can easily slip in.

In the next session, have both spouses report on the degree to which they fulfilled their responsibilities and utilized their privileges. If the couple are *content* with the current terms of their contract and wish to continue adhering to it, they should be encouraged to do so. Both should be asked to express how they feel about their fulfilling the terms of the contract. If one or both partners are *dissatisfied* with their contracts, help them express their feelings using previously learned communication skills. After one spouse describes the feelings and attitudes held, the other partner should reflect these back in an empathic way. The therapist should help the couple refine, revise, or restructure their contract for the coming week. If the couple find the contracting noxious and clearly do not wish to continue with it, they should be allowed to stop the contracting. Before giving up the contracting, ask if they would like to make a completely different contract by starting at the first step of the contracting exercise. A retyped copy of revised contracts should be furnished to the couple together with record sheets. In future sessions, the contract is regularly reviewed, revised, or renegotiated as needed.

After agreeing to a contract and carrying it out at home successfully, the couple are encouraged to negotiate agreements between themselves at home as the need arises. That is, the specifying, empathizing, negotiating, and compromising that are involved in forming a contingency contract may be used as a tool for conflict resolution.

—— • ——

Refreshing changes can come when, through contracting, spouses begin to make direct requests of each other. Instead of innuendos or the pejorative assumptions implicit in prefaces such as "I'm sure you don't want me to do this, but . . ." or "The least you could do is . . . ," the couple begin to ask for their desires "up front" and in positive ways.

Bonnie asked Bob if he'd accompany her to church, an important spiritual and social outlet for her. He said, "I've been to jail once and I've been to church once, and once is enough!" However, he did go to church after Bonnie agreed, in a contract, to give him a weekly massage.

—— • ——

Differences over child management can be ameliorated by contracts. John agreed to spend more time with their daughter if his wife, Sue, would stop putting him down in front of the children. Sue asked him how much time he was willing to spend with their daughter, and he replied, "Five minutes a week." By the end of the therapy, he was spending several hours a week with their daughter spontaneously and enthusiastically.

—— • ——

Don and Rosemary, a couple married for 22 years, came to the group with complaints of growing distance and withdrawal. Don felt that Rosemary no longer demonstrated her love for him, and Rosemary countered by saying that Don rarely discussed family matters with her and either avoided household responsibilities or criticized her for making decisions. After three sessions of specifying and negotiating the terms of an agreement, they signed the following contract:

Don's responsibilities	Don's privileges
To converse with wife 15 minutes a day at a mutually convenient time.	Wife will initiate sex once a week.
To give wife one hour of time alone twice weekly.	To be able to work on hobby twice weekly for one hour each time.

Rosemary's responsibilities	Rosemary's privileges
To express approval for husband's actions once a day.	To be able to make plans for entertainment once a week.
To tell husband that she loves him or to call him "Honey" three times a week.	Husband will complete one household task a week with criteria for satisfactory completion specified in advance.

—— • ——

At each session, ask the couple if conflicts have come up and if they tried to use their contracting skills to resolve them. If they tried and were successful, have them talk about their success. If they tried and failed to resolve the conflict, ask them to try it again during the session. In this way, you can provide feedback and coach them as they go through it, pointing out where they did and did not use the skills properly. Encourage them to try using contracting again during the coming week as conflicts arise and to report back on how it worked. If a couple report that conflicts came up but they did not use contracting for resolution, have them try it during the session while being prompted, coached, and given positive and negative feedback by you as they move through the process.

During the time that the couple are learning to negotiate and monitor contracts, it is often helpful if you call them one or twice during the week. These phone calls can be used to prompt them to adhere to the contract terms and to troubleshoot any problems that may have come up in the process. This is also an opportunity to support and encourage their efforts to use the specifying, requesting, negotiating, and compromising skills to deal with differences and conflicts that may have come up between sessions. In this way, you can help the couple generalize the skills learned during therapy sessions to the home environment. In Table VIII are listed four sample contracts.

TABLE VIII. Contingency Contracts Developed by Four Married Couples

	Contingencies	
Couple	*Responsibilities*	*Privileges*
1 Wife	To greet husband affectionately every day when he comes home from work.	Husband will express his feelings and thoughts to me daily at lunch or after work.
	To plan budget on Sundays at 1 P.M. for half hour.	Husband will give me a massage for 20 minutes once a week.
1 Husband	To express approval for something that wife does well once a week.	Wife will initiate plans for all leisure time on Saturday.

TABLE VIII. (continued)

	Contingencies	
Couple	*Responsibilities*	*Privileges*
	To call wife on phone every night from work between 9:30 and 10:00 P.M.	Wife will be more pleasant in the morning and will fix a breakfast for every two phone calls.
2 Wife	To comply with or refuse a request in a friendly way each day.	Husband will do same.
	To initiate sex once a week.	Husband will tolerate my friends and be positive when discussing them.
2 Husband	To converse with wife on five of seven days for five minutes, each time on a topic of her choice.	Wife will listen to my views on future work and residence plans once a week for 20 minutes.
	To go to church with wife once a month.	Wife will give me a massage every other day for at least 5 minutes for 30 days following church attendance.
3 Wife	To tolerate and forgive husband's mistakes.	Husband will do same.
	To allow husband two hours a week to play with son alone.	Husband will take me to lunch or dancing once a week.
3 Husband	To complete weekly chores without reminders.	Wife will go for pleasure ride in car with me for 30 minutes once a week.
	To give wife advance notice when working late.	Wife will respond in a friendly way when given notice about late working.
	To get car serviced once a week.	Wife will help to plan household repairs and chores.
4 Wife	To clean one room of house to husband's satisfaction each week.	Husband will express approval of work once a day.
	To massage husband three times a week.	Husband will reciprocate.
4 Husband	To ask about wife's feelings one or two times a day.	Wife will tolerate or say something nice about two of my friends.
	To spend three hours a week doing something together with whole family.	Wife will initiate sex three times a week.

SUMMARY OF GUIDELINES FOR CONDUCTING CONTRACTING IN A GROUP FORMAT

1. Begin with a couple who are likely to be cooperative and have success in going through the steps of the contracting exercise scheduled for that session. This provides a further model for other group members.
2. Solicit feedback from other group members on how spouses might make their requests more specific. Have group members comment on the communication skills each partner is using while negotiating and compromising during the session.
3. Cut off any efforts by other group members to railroad a spouse into agreeing with responsibilities or privileges that he/she does not honestly feel can be fulfilled.

REFERENCES

DeRisi, W. J., & Butz, G. *Writing behavioral contracts*. Champaign, Ill.: Research, 1975.

Homme, L. E., Csanyi, A., Gonzales, M., & Rechs, J. *How to use contingency contracting in the classroom*. Champaign, Ill.: Research, 1969.

Stuart, R. B. Behavioral contracting with the families of delinquents. *Journal of Behavior Therapy and Experimental Psychiatry*, 1971, *2*, 1–11.

CHAPTER 7

Ending

The ending of a program of marital therapy or marriage counseling has many of the same elements as the termination of any other kind of therapy. There may be a recurrence of symptoms and an unwillingness to give up the dependent relationship with the therapist. There can be expressions of sadness, separation anxiety, or other emotions just when you expect the greatest improvement. It is important that these trends be recognized for what they are and that they be discussed with the couple without discouragement.

Methods for dealing with termination should include the use of time structure, fading procedures, reinforcement of gains, sharing of sadness, emphasis on what the couples are taking with them, and planning for the future. They take with them new insights, new sources of support, new habits, and new tools for problem solving. The plans for the future may or may not include additional counseling.

TIME STRUCTURE

Setting a time limit for therapy is important as it helps you and the couple to mobilize strengths and come to grips with the goals that have been set. Clients should participate, and milestones like anniversaries, vacations, births, and moving can be incorporated into meaningful planning. Indefinitely long therapy, without logically defined time sequences, is conducive to staying with the past and procrastinating in regard to taking action in the present. If goals are set with no relation to a time structure, some of the incentive to change is missing and the client is robbed of the sense of achievement that comes from accomplishing something within a certain period of time. Time structure can always be revised, but it should never be abandoned. The time structure that was developed in your initial therapeutic contract with the couple in all probability has helped them anticipate the termination from the start so that they have had appropriate expectations and a realistic point of view that have acted as an antidote to their fear of going it alone.

FADING PROCEDURES

Sessions can be shortened and scheduled at longer intervals so that the couple can try their wings and gradually get used to being on their own. This procedure is known as *fading*. For example, after seeing the couple for 8 or 10 weekly sessions, the sessions might be scheduled bimonthly. By spacing the sessions further apart, newly acquired behaviors can be practiced and independently sustained for longer and longer periods of time. Sometimes a planned vacation from therapy for a designated time period can also enhance independence.

Lonnie and Marge were concerned that their cross-country camping trip in their minibus would be a fiasco because it could not be postponed and therefore had to be undertaken when they had been in therapy for only four sessions. When this less-than-ideal timing was reframed as an opportunity to practice a new kind of communication, Lonnie and Marge capitalized on it. They used their third and fourth sessions to air their apprehensions, request support from each other in specific, nondestructive ways, and do some planning for privacy along the way. Marge requested a motel stop every third night. Lonnie would not agree to that but guaranteed an average of every third night. He requested less backseat driving and diligent map-reading. Marge agreed, provided that she received the same courtesy and cooperation while she drove. During their visits with parents, each was to be free to leave his/her spouse with his/her parents for a half-day of individual recreation, for seeing friends, shopping, or whatever. They both also would support each other in front of in-laws, and neither would dis-

cuss the other behind her or his back. This newly established loyalty took away a lot of the dread of the trip. An inconvenient time frame was then turned into an advantage. Lonnie had been in favor of canceling the trip entirely and was glad they had not done so.

—— • ——

A couple can be helped to plan their own refresher or brushup, either after a set time interval or as needed. Marge felt more secure when follow-up appointments were set in advance, so they would not indicate dissatisfaction but would be more associated with "growth" than "need," as she put it.

With the encouragement of the therapist, some couples develop rituals for celebrating their completing marriage counseling as they would their wedding anniversary. Rereading their marital therapy contract and renewing it, a session with you to amend it, or a telephone call or letter to keep you up-to-date on their progress are all helpful follow-up procedures. This kind of planned follow-up is an effective aid in termination. It not only benefits the couple in the consolidation of their gains but also benefits you for research and evaluation purposes.

—— • ——

Mary and Arthur decided on a follow-up appointment six weeks after the termination of therapy, then another after three months. The first follow-up was timed to allow for preparatory planning for Mary's mother's visit, as they both feared a setback at that time. The later appointment was to allow for planning a more rewarding vacation, since the last two had been ruined by bickering and arguing to the point where they couldn't agree on what they wanted to do. They also said they would like to have an annual contact with the therapist—either a three-way telephone conference or an interview, depending on where they were.

REINFORCEMENT

There should be reinforcement of gains all along the way, of course, but especially toward the end of counseling as a way of minimizing anxiety, distress, or feelings of helplessness. By frequently acknowledging the positive changes that have occurred in their actions, attitudes, and feelings, you can help the couple consolidate and strengthen their new interaction patterns. The more reinforcement you give for progress in your clients, the less you will have to deal with termination anxiety and relapses. You also will want to teach the partners to reinforce each other.

—— • ——

Hal and Doreen became reinforcing to each other after they learned what exactly was reinforcing to each of them. Doreen took offense when it was pointed out to her that money was reinforcing to her, as she felt that was inconsistent with her value system. However, she was assured by both Hal and the therapist that they were not viewing this in a moral context but were impressed with what an outstanding manager she was and how she thrived on having concrete data on which to base her excellent planning. Hal had a similar reaction when it was brought out that sex was what reinforced him. He protested that this included physical affection and that he certainly wanted it to be mutual.

Discussion of money embarrassed Hal. He took it as Doreen's putting him down for not earning more. Talk about sex embarrassed her, so they had been using exactly the wrong methods to reinforce each other. It often happens that a partner will assume that what is reinforcing to him/her is also reinforcing to his/her partner. Hal would approach Doreen sexually when what she really wanted for her own security was to know what his take-home pay would be the next week. She would try to give him reassurance by reporting on their savings account when what he really wanted was for her to go to bed with him. Awareness of their needs and their partner's needs increased reciprocity and paved the way for a much happier marriage. As termination neared, the therapist's role was to lend his weight to the positive exchanges already occurring.

—— • ——

Here are some examples of how a therapist can teach married clients to reinforce each other, followed by further reinforcement for their reciprocity:

JIM: Her cooking is improving—it really isn't anywhere near as bad as it used to be.

THERAPIST: How does that feel to you, Joan?

JOAN: Not very good—as if I'd gone from ghastly to not-quite-so-ghastly, but still rotten.

THERAPIST: Would you want to rephrase that more positively, Jim?

JIM: Honey, the chicken dinner you cooked last night was just terrific!

THERAPIST: Aren't you going to respond to that?

JOAN: I'm glad you liked it.

THERAPIST: Jim, is she getting across to you that she appreciated your positive feedback?

JIM: Well, it did sound somewhat perfunctory.

JOAN: *(Trying again.)* Jim, it really pleases me when you praise my cooking, and I especially like it when you don't link it up with what a lousy cook I was for so many years.

JIM: I didn't realize that made you feel so put down.

JOAN: Not so much put down as guilty.

JIM: I had no idea I was making you feel guilty. I think you're practically a gourmet cook now, and I love it.

THERAPIST: That's better. Keep sharing your pleasure with Joan's cooking if you want the gourmet meals to continue.

Another example:

MARGARET: I wanted to tell you that Bert has telephoned each night he's had to work late. It's been just great.

THERAPIST: Did you tell him that?

BERT: No, she didn't. As a matter of fact, I hesitated to call last night because the night before she sounded annoyed that I'd interrupted one of her TV programs.

MARGARET: I just mentioned it. I didn't really mind.

BERT: I don't know. You sound sort of "whiny" over the telephone.

MARGARET: I do not.

THERAPIST: Bert, tell Margaret exactly how you would like her to respond to you on the telephone.

BERT: Could you say you're glad I called? Or ask me how I am?

MARGARET: Aren't you being rather fussy?

THERAPIST: Do you want him to keep calling?

MARGARET: I definitely do. OK, I'll try. I see what you mean. Unless I give a positive response, he'll stop calling. Well, at least I don't bawl you out on the phone the way I used to, do I, Bert?

BERT: No, but . . .

THERAPIST: Why don't you reinforce her for the improvement she has made and then ask for what more you want without any accusation?

BERT: How did you know I was going to accuse her of . . . Oh, OK Margaret, I just love not being bawled out (with a smile) and I'll keep calling when I'm going to be late because I enjoy talking with you on the telephone.

MARGARET: *(Smiling.)* I like to talk with you, too, and I really do like it when you call.

THERAPIST: Now you're on the right track with positive feedback and Warm Fuzzies.

Another example:

JENNIFER: He never says anything good about me. It's nothing but criticize, criticize, criticize.

DAVID: Just this morning I told her I liked her sweater, and she went into a regular diatribe about how she has nothing to wear, the sweater was an old rag, and I didn't care about her. What's the use of trying to pay her a compliment? She's never accepted one in her life.

JENNIFER: Well, I don't call that a compliment, telling me that . . .

THERAPIST: Did you hear, though, that he's discouraged because you rarely accept a compliment? By the way, that's a pretty necklace you're wearing.

JENNIFER: Oh, this is just a . . . Oh, thank you. *(Looking miserable.)*

THERAPIST: Sometimes it's possible to reinforce the intent even if the content isn't acceptable. Could you try to do that?

JENNIFER: You mean from this morning? David, well, I appreciated that you noticed what I was wearing. I really did. Could we talk about my need for new clothes sometime?

DAVID: Sure, and I like it when you acknowledge my interest in your looks. I think you're lovely and you deserve some new clothes.

THERAPIST: Both of you can get what you want and need from each other through positive means.

Another example:

THERAPIST: Well, Joe and Maria, you both seem satisfied now with how your marriage is going.

JOE: Yes, she's finally doing her duty as a wife.

THERAPIST: Maria?

MARIA: I do not like your putting it that way, Joe. We're both being responsible, and we need to keep giving each other Warm Fuzzies to keep it going.

JOE: That's right. You're doing a lot more than your duty, and so am I for that matter. Don't you think so?

MARIA: I sure do. I'm really happy that you're helping me with the kids.

THERAPIST: That's great, Joe. And how do you feel now about Maria's going to school?

JOE: As long as she keeps doing things with me and with the family and isn't studying all the time, it's OK with me. I've never told her this, but I'm really proud of her.

THERAPIST: Why don't you tell her?

JOE: You know, don't you, Maria, that I'm proud of you—going to school and all?

MARIA: No, I didn't know, and thank you for telling me. It makes me very happy. I thought you resented my going to school.

JOE: I did—but not anymore.

THERAPIST: Why not?

JOE: Maria talks to me more now. She's not turning away from me, so I'm not jealous of her schoolwork anymore.

THERAPIST: It's important that you keep telling her that you appreciate her not turning away and that you are proud of her, isn't it?

JOE: And that she keeps thanking me for helping with the kids.

MARIA: Right, Joe, if you weren't cooperating, I couldn't possibly go to school. You know that. And it's wonderful for the kids to have you with them more.

JOE: You're a good wife.

By the time of termination, each client should have a deepened awareness of the importance of positive reciprocity and a larger repertoire of ways of giving PLEASES to the partner and of ways of asking for PLEASES. Giving and getting PLEASES with one's partner makes it easier to give PLEASES to oneself. Reciprocity and self-reinforcement both raise self-esteem as they improve marital satisfaction.

SHARING SADNESS AT SAYING GOOD-BYE

There can be real pain at parting, and some of your clients will attempt to turn the therapeutic relationship into a personal and social one as a means of prolonging it. You will want to say good-bye without denying the finality of the ending, while at the same time leaving the door open for future counseling or for structured follow-up as indicated. There may be resistance to "getting well" because it signifies the end of your support, so you will want to express your confidence in your clients and their continued growth.

WHAT THEY TAKE WITH THEM

The positive side of ending—the compensation for the loss—is what the couple have attained that will remain with them. When they say good-bye to you, they should recognize that they are taking away something under their belts. During the counseling process, they have developed more insight into their responsibilities for the relationship and are less likely to blame their partners for marital distress. They have grasped the concept of reciprocity; they know that what they derive from their marriage is inextricably linked with what they put into it. This knowledge has come from more than just advice and discussion on an intellectual level: they have practiced it, lived it, and experienced it to the point where they are highly motivated to keep on applying it to their daily lives. You will want to encourage them to hang onto these newly acquired insights and skills.

One way of building in durability for their progress is to anticipate with them realistic but hypothetical problems that might occur in the future and to ask them how they would resolve them with no therapist around to help. You might question them by asking, "Suppose that your grandmother asked to come and live with you?"; or "What if you discovered a marijuana plant growing in Adrienne's closet?"; or "What will happen if Tom gets a six-month layoff from work?"; or "What if Sue suffers a relapse and gets seriously depressed again?" Ask them how they would react. Would they panic? Explore with them whether they would let new stresses force them back into the old, aversive patterns of behavior. Would they return to unilateral actions with no allowance for mutual decision-making, blame, or withdrawal? Or are their new reaction patterns and problem-solving behaviors firmly enough established for the couple to apply them? Under what circumstances would they consider returning to therapy? What steps would they take first prior to resorting to professional help? Helping the couple go through some anticipated problem solving is like putting money in the bank for coping with future conflicts.

NEW INTERACTION PATTERNS

Couples' investments in counseling will have yielded new patterns of interaction in their marriages and lives. Core symbols may be reaffirmed or new ones developed. They may have made new friends in their recreation as individuals or as a couple. For example, Mary and Arthur's contract (see Table IX) included his going to church with her and her going camping with him. Relationships made at church turned out to be sources of emotional support, and camping friends were added to their social network.

During the termination process, you should recognize and reinforce the new habits that have been learned and emphasize the need to practice them. Any new behavior, especially a communication skill, has to be repeated over and over again for the couple to attain competence and comfort. If a better relationship with the children is one of the outcomes of treatment, then you will want to stress the importance of continuing to practice the improved parent–child interactions—whether a program for the distribution of household chores, parents' getting together on discipline in private and supporting each other in front of the children, or more attention given to family recreation.

Help the marital partners become aware of what helped and how it helped. Then, individualized problem-solving strategies can be used both preventively and remedially in the future. Marriages never remain the same. They are in a continuing process of growth or deterioration.

TABLE IX. Marital Contract Agreed Upon by Mary and Arthur Peabody

Mary	
Responsibilities	*Privileges*
1. Mary will spend a minimum of one hour each pay day going over the bills and the budget.	1. Mary may use up to 20% of her earnings for baby-sitting fees and for a cleaning woman.
2. Mary will initiate sex at least once a week.	2. Arthur will give Mary a back and shoulder rub at least once a week.
3. Arthur can bring guests home for dinner once every two weeks, provided he gives Mary two hours' notice and helps clean up the house afterwards.	3. Arthur will go for walks with Mary amounting to one hour of time over the course of a month.
Arthur	
Responsibilities	*Privileges*
1. Arthur will go to at least two church events of *his* choice each month. They can be services or socials.	1. Mary will help Arthur with yard work at least one hour per week.
2. Arthur will take Mary out to dinner once a week.	2. Mary will prepare a favorite meal of Arthur's once a week (on the weekend).
3. Arthur will baby-sit at least two hours per week.	3. Mary will organize a family picnic once a month.

Only practice will ensure that the new skills that the couples have worked so hard to learn and apply will become a permanent part of their marriage.

—— • ——

Mary and Arthur reported that executive sessions were incorporated as part of their lifestyle and that they have every intention of keeping it that way. In one executive session, when they were discussing their daughter Lisa's need for orthodontia, Mary was hell-bent to have Lisa's teeth straightened immediately. On the other hand, Arthur wanted to wait until they had some money saved. Mary said, "I heard Arthur say, 'Let's go to the dentist and talk it over,' instead of my misinterpreting that he was trying to buck me." Arthur said, "I heard Mary's complaints about Lisa's teeth—knowing I just had to reflect back was a relief. I finally realized she wasn't demanding a final decision but rather wanted me to listen and hear her. It's really made a difference."

One of the later executive sessions had as its focus how much longer they needed to continue in marital therapy. Arthur expressed his financial concerns and Mary her fears that her headaches would return, but not until she had first reassured him of her intention to continue their financial conferences and to keep within the budget. Then, she requested that if her headaches recurred, they could come back to the therapist. Arthur heard this and was supportive. These sessions led to some compromising, such as their mutual decision to have six-week and then three-month follow-up sessions timed to help with Mary's mother's visit and their own vacation plans.

—— • ——

The tools that the couples have acquired need to be identified in such a way that the couples see that these tools can replace the therapy. When marital communication breaks down, tracking Warm Fuzzies can be reinstituted, executive sessions can be scheduled to reopen communication and deescalate quarrels. As controversial issues arise, signaling the need for new compromises, contracts can be renegotiated and new agreements reached. In addition to their contract, a couple may be encouraged to take on more long-term homework assignments—ones that are not going to be handed in—as another way to replace therapy.

FUTURE PLANNING

At the point of termination, there should be full and free discussion of further needs for the couple. Appropriate referrals can be made for additional help, such as a course in parenting skills, a women's assertiveness-training group, or family therapy. When sexual problems remain even after verbal communication and the exchange of PLEASES are mutually satisfactory, you may want to refer the couple for sex therapy. If no referral for additional work is indicated, you can say good-bye while allowing for subsequent follow-up contacts either scheduled or on a looser, "as needed" basis. Setbacks before, during, and after termination should not be allowed to affect the couple seriously, since brief interactions can often help get communication back on the track. Good-byes with future planning lessen the finality and therefore the anxiety about ending. In most cases, the door you leave open will not be entered by your clients; however, it will sustain them and enable them to return to you without losing face when they again need your assistance.

EVALUATION

Before the end of the final session, the "Marital Adjustment Test" should be completed. The results, which almost always indicate marked improvement, should be reviewed and shared to the extent that you feel would be helpful. A copy of the "Marital Adjustment Test" and a "Client Satisfaction Questionnaire" are in the "Client's Workbook." Improvements in score on the posttest provide another opportunity to give reinforcement to the couple. Evaluative feedback from the couple's questionnaires and their verbal comments can also help you plan improvements in your treatment procedures and your future practice of marital therapy. As gains are celebrated, new long-term goals need to be set so that the ending of therapy is also a new beginning—the beginning of a more satisfying phase of each couple's married life.

ENDING GROUP MARITAL THERAPY

Termination of married couples' groups has the same elements as terminating treatment with a couple. Time structure and fading procedures are especially helpful for couples in groups. The group can be prompted to reach a consensus about a refresher session or a reunion six months or a year later. Planned follow-ups benefit the couples in helping them sustain their gains and also enable the therapist to evaluate longer-term outcomes. Follow-up sessions can take the form of marathons or minimarathons, such as a half-day or a full evening.

Follow-up sessions are reinforcing in many ways. For you, the counselor, and for the participants, a reunion is an occasion based on growth. The emphasis is on positive changes in the marriage and on the generalization of the gains made during marital therapy. The couples use these sessions to assure themselves that things are still OK, to offer reinforcement if they are, and to offer help if they are not. Modeling provides mutual assistance because the couples are eager to share which of their new problem-solving procedures were brought into play and how they worked.

—— • ——

At one such reunion, Larry described a bitter argument that he and Joan had had after a party. It had been their first fight since the end of the married couples' workshop. It had taken them both somewhat by surprise and had shaken them up, as they had felt that they had gotten beyond that sort of destructive display of anger. Even an ice cream break had not helped. He hadn't felt that an executive session would either, at that point, so he had decided he would try a love day. He was obviously proud of his strategy as he recounted how he had done the laundry, had spoken to his mother-in-law on the telephone, and had reviewed all the contract items to refresh his mind as to what was particularly reinforcing to Joan. He complimented her on her cooking, listened to her attentively, let her select the TV programs, took out the garbage, and told her she looked beautiful. Joan laughed and said, "It took me awhile to catch on, but even when I did, it was far better than an apology. His giving me all those PLEASES *was just what I needed to soften me up so I could handle an executive session. Before the marital group, I would have continued to punish him and nothing would have been resolved. During the executive session, we both knew how to confront the problem without trying to destroy each other. I told him how hurt I had felt when he neglected me at the party and flirted with my girlfriend. Now I can own up to my feelings instead of telling him he was an insensitive bastard, the way I used to. He listened and told me what they'd been talking about. We really worked it out."*

—— • ——

Don said he and his wife, Francie, had resorted to another set of strategies, maybe because their backsliding took another form. They just seemed to be growing apart again, which is what had brought them to marriage counseling in the first place. As he thought about the flatness that was returning to the relationship, he remem-

bered how impressed he had been by the group's emphasis on greetings after coming home from work. One day after work, he was heading straight to the refrigerator for a beer with hardly a "Hi" when he caught himself, retraced his steps, and deliberately took his wife in his arms. After a hug, he asked her if she'd like to go out for dinner. Several times, he went out of his way to get the evening off to a good start. "And, wow," he added, "has it paid off!" He described how when the tone was set, even if they each did go off and do their own thing for most of the evening, there was a different atmosphere in the house: quiet companionship or comfortable awareness of the other's presence instead of feelings of isolation. Francie said, "And don't forget the mornings. I'm no longer quite the zombie I was. Since Don is making such an effort when he comes home tired at night, I'm trying to be more pleasant in the morning. I used to be one of those don't-dare-speak-to-me-till-I've-had-my-coffee types, but I'm getting over that." Don thanked her for acknowledging his efforts and said he really appreciated her early morning pleasantness.

—— • ——

Participants in groups have difficulty saying good-bye to you, the therapist, and also to each other. The group has become part of their support system. Some groups wish to continue to meet socially, independent of the therapist. Friendships occasionally are made that outlast the life of the group. This has long been frowned upon in traditional therapy, but in our experience, we have found these social connections a constructive supplement to the therapy experience. Even when members go out for coffee after group sessions, issues of significance discussed among the members always get back to the group meetings. Thus, fear of diluting the group experience is unfounded.

The group format facilitates the use of reunions for therapeutic purposes. Couples come prepared with questions that they want to raise with the group. They come expecting to give and get feedback and to get help in solving old or new problems. One couple, Les and Janice, returned with an old problem—her jealousy—taking a new form. Les was socializing Friday evenings with his fellow narcotics agents, and Janice was feeling jealous, angry, and left out, especially when she heard indirectly that some of the wives were being included. Les said that she could come occasionally but that he wanted to be free to join his colleagues spontaneously without feeling that he had to arrange for her to make the 50-minute ride to come every time. The group leader was about to set up an executive session with modeling and coaching when Joan interjected, "Janice, you and Les are talking that problem to death. Why beat a dead horse? I've heard you say many times that you never had time to go shopping with your daughter or get your hair done. This is your golden opportunity. I think you'd feel better if you just did your own thing Friday nights instead of staying home and brooding about being left out." Janice said that she'd try it but that she didn't think it would diminish her jealous feelings. This opened up the whole subject of jealousy, which had not been covered adequately during the workshop. Several participants shared their experiences and what worked for them. Some had found that just acknowledging that they felt jealous and giving themselves permission to be jealous instead of chastising themselves for it was all that they needed. Gus felt it necessary to make requests for reassurance, then to contract on how much outside socializing as individuals would be acceptable to him and to his wife. There was a consensus that jealousy stems from feelings of insecurity and that they are natural feelings to have at times. The question arose of how much to attend to these feelings, as they could be blown up out of proportion. Janice felt that the discussion had been helpful to her in getting a perspective on the problem. She said that she was not going to let it get out of hand this time. Les immediately reinforced her for this by saying that if she could take those occasional Friday nights in her stride, he'd see that their Saturday nights were special. Janice had accepted help from Joan and other group members and did not need the therapist's suggestion to tackle the problem in another way.

Sometimes flare-ups of marital discord just before termination can be disconcerting and even threatening to your own sense of success or competency as a therapist. Madge and Chris needed to be referred for divorce counseling after what had seemed a relatively successful course of marital therapy. Six months later, they attempted reconciliation and reapplied for marital therapy. They attended a series of group sessions before they felt that they had the requisite communication skills to feel comfortable about continuing their marriage. Treatment strategies need to be kept flexible, as marriage relationships can be in an almost constant state of flux, and readiness for various kinds of interventions is not always predictable.

When the subject of termination is taken up in a group, there may be those who are not ready and who need more help. Some may want to recycle and participate in another group, while others might want to go into conjoint therapy. New courses of treatment with new goals and new time frames can be developed. Feedback from test results can be used along with verbal feedback as an opportunity to reinforce the couples on their progress and to reinforce you, the therapist, on the job you have done. If you broaden your skills to include group marital therapy, you will be advancing your know-how and facilitating your professional growth.

CHAPTER 8

Solving Special Problems

Throughout this guide we have described a variety of techniques or strategies for treating troubled relationships. Our experience and research have repeatedly demonstrated their effectiveness. However, knowing what couples need to do is only a beginning for the therapist. How do you get couples to engage in the activities that you feel will lead to an enhanced relationship? How can you ensure that couples carry out homework assignments that will promote the maintenance of the communication techniques they are acquiring in the therapy? How do you deal with problem situations that occur during treatment and may threaten positive outcomes or hinder the couple's progress?

Behaviorally oriented therapists have often been criticized for assuming that rational, task- and data-oriented approaches will be openly received by couples experiencing relationship dysfunctions. In fact, resistance to behavioral interventions does occur and must be dealt with if treatment is to succeed. This chapter provides suggestions for handling clients' resistances to goal setting and to role playing and homework assignments. A section is included on dealing with special problems, such as a spouse's dropping out of treatment, dealing with unexpected outbursts, and including unwed couples in married couples' groups.

OVERCOMING RESISTANCE TO BEHAVIORAL GOALS

When we speak of *resistance* to a behavioral or learning approach, we mean noncooperation with the therapist's efforts to change behavior. When resistance to the procedures described in this guide occurs, it typically revolves around two types of issues:

1. Resistance to the goals of the behavioral approach
2. Resistance to some of the specific techniques and approaches employed

As you may remember, the goals of behavioral marital therapy are to have couples (1) increase their positively reinforcing exchanges; (2) decrease their aversive interchanges; and (3) acquire the communication and problem-solving skills needed to negotiate changes in their relationship.

While most couples perceive these goals as being important areas to work on and relevant to their problems, some do not. The following monologue by an upset husband illustrates this type of resistance:

> I didn't come here to learn how to please, listen to, and talk more understandably with my wife. I came because I'm sick and tired of her constant nagging about everything she's unhappy about. If she doesn't watch it, I'm going to hit her again or leave and have another affair. I want you to tell me why she's like that and get her to stop.

Frequently, resistance to the general goals of this behaviorally oriented approach to therapy can be overcome by the following activities.

ORIENTATION AND RATIONALE

Carefully orient the couple to the treatment procedures that will be employed. The rationale that you use should be easily understood and absorbed by the couple. As the therapist, you might, for example, briefly explain and demonstrate the difference between pleasing exchanges and aversive exchanges. The couple might then be drawn into a brief discussion of the typical consequences following positive and negative exchanges. Similarly, the goals behind teaching effective communication, listening, and negotiation skills should be clearly explained and illustrated. Most couples experiencing discord readily

when we're calm and relaxed, but it's impossible for me to talk with him when he's angry, and he's not angry today.

HUSBAND: Furthermore, as you well know, some of our problems concern sex. You can't really expect us to practice that with you present.

A couple's resistance to behavioral rehearsal that stems from feelings that the activity is artificial or from shyness can typically be overcome in the following manner.

First, you might rehearse the situation for one or both spouses while they simply observe. Then ask the partners to critique, revise, and elaborate on your performance to make the situation more real. Use their feedback to improve your second attempt at the scene. After again eliciting feedback, you might comment on the situation's emotional realness for you and suggest that it would be even more real if the spouses now tried it themselves. You might also briefly note that the couple's feedback was helpful and that you would be happy to provide similar feedback when they try it.

A second approach you might use is to ignore the resistant verbalizations and ask the client to describe in concrete, graphic details what happens *in vivo* during the problem situation. As the client does this, you subtly slip into role playing. For example, "When he said you were only interested in the children, you said ______." You then follow the client's response with a response that her husband might make. After two or three exchanges, you have, in fact, engaged the client in a role-play situation with you. Typically, clients laugh at this point and say that it did feel somewhat real and was not that difficult to do.

A third approach that can be used is to role-play the scene with a co-therapist and have one or both spouses serve as doubles or auxiliary egos for the therapists. As the therapist provides sufficient opportunity for the clients to become more and more involved, it is only a small step to engage the clients directly in the rehearsal.

A fourth option is to have a resistant client take the role of a target other than himself or herself. When a spouse who is reluctant to rehearse takes the partner's part, this is called *role reversal*. This enables the reluctant spouse to get involved in a role that is not quite as personally threatening as his or her own role. If you are working with a married couples group, you can also have the reluctant client help his or her fellow group members by taking a role in one of the other couple's scenes.

A fifth alternative is to physically and persistently prompt resistant clients to get up and move into the scene with gentle tugs, pats or pressure on the back, or hand holding while you give firm, repeated verbal prompts to "give it a try." Your physical touch and proximity make it more difficult for clients to decline your invitation to participate. At the same time, your close proximity reassures the clients of your support and of your being with them in the scene.

Lastly, you may acknowledge the resistant client's feelings, inhibitions, anxieties, and reasons for not wanting to participate *without* elaborate psychological interpretations, *without* cajoling, and *without* excessive reassurance. After brief acknowledgment, *prompt* the client toward an attainable approximation to role playing. You might, for example, use the third or fourth alternative previously described as the client's first step in this direction.

RESISTANCE TO BEHAVIORAL REHEARSAL IN GROUP MARITAL THERAPY

One of the main advantages of working with a group of couples is the availability of additional options to overcoming resistances to behavioral rehearsal. While the group setting may increase resistances due to shyness, most of the other types of resistance can be more easily overcome by utilizing the group process.

Enthusiasm begets enthusiasm. Therefore, one of the first things to do in a group setting to overcome resistance to role playing is to begin with the most enthusiastic couple. A veteran couple who have successfully participated in role playing would be good participants to begin with. Enthusiastic veteran clients usually provide good models for more resistant clients.

A second option, if you have an open-ended group, is to allow resistant and new clients simply to observe during the first one or two sessions. This motivates them to participate because they see the activities that are modeled for them as helpful, meaningful, and enjoyable. Additionally, the therapist's attention and comments given to actively participating couples are powerful reinforcers that nonparticipating couples are deprived of.

Third, ask resistant clients to give verbal suggestions and feedback to other participating members as approximations to active involvement. After two or three suggestions, you may want to ask these clients to demonstrate their suggestions for the participating clients, thereby shaping an approximation to their rehearsing a scene in their own marriage.

In addition to shaping more active participation in the group through these activities, you may want initially to have a resistant couple rehearse easier scenes. The couple might be prompted to try a short, nonthreatening scene without a heavy personal loading. Such scenes include introducing oneself to others in the group or giving one piece of information about oneself to another group member.

A fifth approach to dealing with clients' resistance to role playing in the group situation is to ask other group members to talk about how they overcame their resistances and shyness. Typically, experienced clients say that they had similar reservations but that they have found the behavioral rehearsals to be enjoyable and very helpful.

RESISTANCE TO HOMEWORK

Homework assignments are given to couples at each session. Homework involves having them practice specific skills that they have rehearsed during the session on a regular basis at home. Homework completion by couples is important in helping them consolidate and generalize skills to their home environment. It has been our experience that couples who regularly complete their homework assignments show greater improvements in their relationship than couples who do not. For this reason, the therapist needs to have a few ideas about how to facilitate homework completion by couples. Below are several common reasons for noncompletion of homework and some solutions that we have found useful in dealing with this problem.

One reason for noncompletion of homework assignments that you may consider is the possibility that the couple have not learned the skill adequately during the therapy session. Having them rehearse it some more under the therapist's supervision will alleviate this problem. Lack of skill acquisition is more likely to be a problem as the couples move into more complex and emotionally loaded areas, such as executive sessions on negative feelings.

A second reason that comes up is "we keep forgetting." This often happens when each spouse is placing the responsibility for initiating the homework on the other. Having them decide during the session who will be responsible for reminding the other of homework or having them place prompts in a conspicuous place sometimes helps.

The recording forms used in the "Catch Your Spouse Doing Something Nice" exercise, the behavior cards from the "Family Happiness Index," and the "Contract Fulfillment Record" are all useful prompts for homework completion. However, to be optimally useful, the recording forms must list specific, reasonable, and limited behaviors. For example, we have found that some couples experience difficulty in filling in the blanks on the behavior cards from the "Family Happiness Index" that call for the specification of what, where, when, and how often a new pleasing event should occur in the upcoming week. Two types of problems typically arise: either too great a change is requested or offered, or one or more of the elements of the behavior are left vague or ambiguous. The following example illustrates both of these problems.

— • —

For a long time Mary Peabody had wanted her husband Arthur's help in caring for the children in the evening. Specifically, she wanted him to keep their older daughter, Lisa, occupied while she got the baby ready for bed. Therefore, she selected a card from the "Care of Children" section of the "Family Happiness Index," which requested that her spouse read a story to the children. She completed the card as follows:

For: Arthur Peabody
Read a story to the children
Which One(s): Lisa
When or How Often: every evening

Since Arthur was not in the habit of reading to Lisa and the "when" was specified as "every evening," it was not likely that he would be able to make such a large change in his typical routine. Furthermore, even if he did read to Lisa every evening, there was no guarantee that Mary's objective of keeping Lisa occupied while she got the baby ready for bed would be satisfied. After raising some questions with the Peabodys as to the feasibility of asking for such a large change and the uncertainty of the "when" dimension, the request was changed to the following:

For: Arthur Peabody
Read a story to the children
Which One(s): Lisa
When or How Often: Monday and Wednesday between 6:45 and 7:15 (while the baby is being made ready for bed)

Arthur was much more positive about completing this homework assignment since the request was clearly stated and did not involve as much time.

— • —

It is also helpful to call, or have a secretary call, couples during the week to see how they are doing on their homework. This acts as a prompt to the couples and further stresses the importance of their completing their homework assignments. This call can also serve as a reminder and confirmation for the time and date of the next session. Failure to attend scheduled appointments, or no-shows, range up to 50% in many mental health settings. A brief call to remind clients of their appointment has been shown to reduce the percentage of no-shows to between 15% and 20% of scheduled appointments; thus, tremendous cost savings are made with little added expense. Our experience has been that such prompts also increase the completion of homework assignments.

A third reason that couples sometimes do not do their homework is that they report that the assignments feel mechanical and unspontaneous. This usually occurs after initial sessions and has to do with the giving, acknowledging, and charting of PLEASES. Encourage the couple to continue their efforts, emphasizing that it usually takes time for warm feelings to accompany the actions of giving and receiving PLEASES. Over time, the mechanical aspects will be replaced by more spontaneous and warm feelings.

A problem that sometimes occurs is that one spouse is completing homework assignments and initiating assignments to be done conjointly, but the other is not completing assignments or responding to the initiatives of the first spouse. If this occurs, the therapist should encourage the spouse who is doing the homework to express feelings of hurt and anger in direct ways, using communication skills. Continue to reinforce the "martyred" spouse's constructive efforts and refocus the couple on *positive changes that have occurred* in their relationship.

In general, some guidelines for dealing with noncompletion of homework are:

1. Stress the reasons for the importance of the homework. Explain that the couples will get out of the therapy only what they put into it.
2. Regularly review homework assignments and give time and attention to the completed assignments rather than to the excuses for uncompleted assignments.
3. When an assignment is given and the couple has rehearsed it in the session, help them specify when, where, and how often they will practice it at home.
4. Call the couple or have a secretary prompt them by phone between sessions.

DROPOUTS

One serious problem that may arise occurs when one spouse decides to drop out of therapy. When a partner drops out, it can have a traumatic impact on the partner who has the desire to continue in counseling. If the withdrawal occurs in a group situation, it can be a disruptive factor and be anxiety-arousing to the other members. Questions will be raised about why the person or the couple left, whether rejection by the therapist is involved, and whether the methods really work at all. What action you take will depend, of course, on your knowledge of the dropout and the situational context. You will want to review and use the part of Chapter 2 that deals with involving the reluctant partner. Perhaps group pressure will encourage the potential dropout to remain. Individual sessions with you may serve to remotivate the person. If a couple feel that their problems are just too different from those of the rest of the group, you may plan to see them as a couple instead of in the group setting. Sometimes one partner will wish to continue alone in a married-couples group, but this is rarely advisable because it leads to discussion about the absent partner that is one-sided, can be unfair, and can degenerate into scapegoating and gossiping. It is better to refer the remaining partner to another kind of therapy group. If one partner drops out of couple counseling, the remaining partner can be assured that individual therapy can be helpful even if the most needful partner is not the one who elects to remain in treatment. The dropout may eventually return if the remaining spouse continues to attend therapy and demonstrates commitment to working on the relationship. A dropout may wish to be seen individually for a period of time for problems that are unrelated to the marriage but that need to be resolved before marital therapy can be properly utilized.

DEALING WITH OUTBURSTS AND CONFLICT

Occasionally, hysterical outbursts, embarrassing comments, surprising revelations, and frightening and anxiety-producing behaviors will occur during a session. Sometimes a spouse may come to a session intoxicated or in the midst of a psychotic decompensation. As a therapist, and particularly as the leader of a couples group, you must have some guidelines for handling these kinds of situations when they arise.

The best way to avoid hysterical outbursts, embarrassment, and other obstructions to the therapy process is through preventive action. Five steps that can be taken to avoid such debacles are:

1. Careful screening and selection of patients for marital therapy
2. Establishing firm and consistent ground rules
3. Making sure that the therapy session is a positive experience for both partners
4. Involving a co-leader
5. Developing backup resources

As for screening, the "sore thumb" principle pointed out in Chapter 2 is expedient when selecting couples compatible in a marital group. If you should have a couple who are at each other's throats to the extent that you cannot get a word in edgewise or who refuse to curtail their mutual hurling of insults and accusations, tell them immediately that you will see them individually. Do not hesitate to be firm and directive when the interaction between the partners is destructively nonstop. Don't apologize or even explain. Stand up and lead one or both of the recriminating partners to the door. Crisis intervention has taught us that sometimes, by distancing antagonists through an immediate *time out*, deescalation and conflict resolution can proceed. Time out can be seen as first aid until more definitive communication skills can be brought into play. When you then see each partner individually, you will be in a better position to evaluate the need for prerequisite or supplementary therapies and the readiness of each for marital therapy. It is up to you to determine the treatment of choice, and if either partner has so little control that "listening" is not possible, then you may choose to recommend individual therapy with marriage counseling as a later goal.

Ground rules should include confidentiality, punctuality, regular attendance, and sobriety during sessions. If one or both partners should arrive under the influence of alcohol or drugs, discontinue the session at once. Explain to both that communication training doesn't work when a partner is drunk, in an uncontrollable rage, sulking, or out of it for any other reason, and that it is better to postpone attempts at serious discussion rather than be sucked into a destructive encounter or be manipulated by aversive behavior. The ground rules may well be tested, so stand your ground, comfortable in the knowledge that if the clients cannot accept these minimal limits, then they are not now sufficiently motivated to benefit from this form of treatment. Of course, you remain available to the responsible partner and leave the door open for the reluctant partner as well.

One way of avoiding angry explosions and hysterical outbursts is to make sure that each therapy session is a positive encounter for *both* partners. Remember that many couples find it easier to separate and divorce rather than face the painfulness of trying to deal with their mutual problems. To keep the sessions positive, we have found that it's important to attend to and quickly intervene if the following ground rules are violated during a session.

First, we are alert for below-the-belt comments. These are comments that may be honest but that deal with particularly sensitive personal issues and often concern something that can't be changed. Buddha said, "Before man speaks he should ask himself these questions: Is it true? Is it necessary? Is it timely?" A spouse who drops a bombshell about a previous affair or about something that can't be changed under the guise of "I'm only being honest!" is in fact punishing his/her partner. Measured honesty about things that can be changed helps to provide a positive atmosphere.

Second, arguments that arise during a session need not be resolved by someone's winning. We typically intervene in arguments to assist each spouse in stating and clarifying his or her position and feeling about the issue at hand. We also use the executive session, reflecting-back format to make sure that the positions and feelings of one spouse are understood and accurately received by the other. We try to move the battling spouses beyond the argument toward making requests for constructive behavior change. Dwelling on who was right and who was wrong is counterproductive. For example, Mary Peabody might condemn her husband Arthur by saying, "You're a lousy father! You don't care about our children!" This outburst would very likely lead to an argument. By intervening and using the executive session format, the couple is instructed and coached to make feeling statements followed by a positive request, such as "Could we find some ways for you to spend more time with our daughter?" Analyzing couples' argument strategies focuses everyone's time and attention on negative aspects of the relationship, thus strengthening the problem and often making the session a negative experience. It's easier, and we believe more productive, simply to acknowledge that people will inevitably get angry about a variety of things; therefore, it's important to learn how to stop arguments quickly and work toward conflict management.

Making sure that each participant receives some positive feedback based on her or his performance, completed homework, and positive suggestions will also preempt destructive interchanges. Mental health workers who have observed demonstrations of this approach to marital therapy have frequently commented that the process seems enjoyable for couples and therapists alike. Keeping the atmosphere positive helps couples remain motivated, involved, and oriented toward improving their relationship rather than worried about protecting themselves from further pain.

If destructive behavior in a session becomes dangerous to the client or others, then you will have to use your own best judgment about whether to involve the police or some other backup resource. If there is a crisis or emergency team in your area and you are the only therapist, you may want to use them as a backup in the event of an emergency. You will feel more comfortable if you check out what services are available, under what circumstances they may be called on, and if you have the appropriate telephone numbers handy. The chances are that you will never have occasion to use them. But if you are prepared, you will never be sorry. If you are not prepared, there is that remote possibility that you will be caught without knowing what to do or where to turn. Problems rarely escalate to dangerous levels if good preventive steps are taken early in the therapy.

The many benefits of co-leadership in a marital group have been mentioned elsewhere, but one of the most helpful aspects is having an available therapist to take care of a participant who is decompensating, in crisis, or otherwise overly disruptive. Sometimes just removing such a client and sitting with him/her is enough. Even this measure should be used sparingly because as many problems as possible should be handled in the context of the group. But if a single participant's behavior is interfering with the progress of the other participants, it is best to invite that person for a brief time out.

UNWED COUPLES

A special situation that may occur in marriage counseling involves unwed couples. Since the beginning of the 1970s, more and more couples who live together are troubled enough about their relationships to seek the assistance of marriage therapists. Cohabitation has become a stage of courtship, often substituting for going steady or an engagement. Couples are also increasingly choosing to live together semipermanently, with strong commitments for sustaining the relationship but without the formal marriage vows. The basic problems of cohabitating couples seem to be much like those of married couples. Cohabitating couples often can't communicate their feelings of tenderness and anger with one another, have difficulty establishing optimal conditions of warmth and closeness, and find it difficult to set joint priorities, negotiate compromises, and deal with conflict. However, a few problem dimensions should be noted and evaluated during the screening process for unwed couples if they are to be involved in marital therapy. If these dimensions are not identified, the unwed couple may feel that their concerns are not being acknowledged and that the therapy is inappropriate to their needs. On the other hand, in a group, married members might resent the unwed couple's participation or belittle their problems because they "aren't really married anyway."

You will want to attend to certain issues during the screening process to ascertain if an unwed couple can benefit from therapy or fit into a marital group. Are the unwed couple contemplating marriage and seeking a premarital checkup to see if they're right for each other? Assessment of the couple's communication skills, negotiation skills, recreational patterns, maturity, and reasons for getting married may be all that is desired or required. Eight to ten sessions of marital therapy that build skills in deficient couples might be inappropriate for such a couple.

Are the couple experiencing insecurity from living together that stems from basic fears of abandonment and uncertainty about closeness? In the screening procedures described earlier (Chapter 2), the couples are asked to make a commitment to stay together until the conclusion of the group. The unwed couple may never have clearly established any type of commitment to stay together other than to "take one day at a time." For such couples, even small problems seem very destructive, as illustrated by the following unwed woman's comment: "These things wouldn't bother me if I were married, since I'd know that minor irritations would ride out their normal course and we'd still be together."

For an unwed couple experiencing insecurity, the negotiation and contracting skills described in this guide would probably be very helpful and may be all that they need.

Some unwed couples may be using your services as a way of calling their partner's bluff. That is, "We have too many problems to get married. Okay, let's work out the problems by going to this group or seeing the marriage counselor." If this is the case, you may want to clarify this issue with the couple before you begin a series of sessions or include them in a group. You also might want to help them establish criteria for determining the level of problem resolution that would bring readiness to make a decision to marry. It is important for the couple to understand that a problem-free relationship isn't necessary for marriage.

A fourth consideration to keep in mind when considering an unwed couple's inclusion in a group revolves around the moral standards of the married couples. Learning to deal effectively with parents and in-laws following marriage is a trying and difficult experience for many couples. This problem is frequently exacerbated for unwed couples by parents who are pressuring them to get married because they view the present arrangement as "living in sin." If such issues are the precipitating cause of the unwed couple's seeking your assistance, placing them in a group with married couples who hold attitudes similar to the couple's parents may result in the unwed couple's being the unfortunate object of the married couples' disapproval. This might be fine if the objectives of the group were to change attitudes, increase the couples' acceptance of other couples, and discuss the changing mores of society. However, these are not the objectives of behavioral marital therapy. It might be preferable to work with unwed couples who are experiencing difficulty in dealing with their parents and in-laws outside of a group of married couples. One focus might then be on helping the unwed couple to effectively express their feelings about their living relationship to their parents.

Undoubtedly, there will be other special problems that you will be faced with while doing marital therapy. You might consider the following strategies to deal with problem situations in your work:

1. Careful screening to ensure that the procedures are appropriate for the couple
2. Providing the couple with a thorough orientation and rationale regarding the expectations, procedures, and goals of this approach
3. Anticipating problems before they occur and developing a repertoire of alternative strategies to deal with them if they occur
4. Keeping the couple or the group focused on positive gains and forward progress rather than on failures, problems, and disappointments

CHAPTER 9

Summary

Marital therapy in this handbook is presented as a positive approach to helping troubled relationships. The approach is equally applicable to couples experiencing severe conflict and strain and to those for whom the grind of daily routine and habit have dulled the luster of attachment and attraction. The key concept in marital therapy is communication training. Communication includes accurate and empathic listening as well as the direct and constructive expression of feelings. Effective communication pervades and mediates all aspects of married life: recreation, socializing, child management, money and budgeting, household chores, affection and sex, companionship, and conflict resolution. In this summary, we shall briefly review the contents of each of the chapters with an emphasis on the clinical, practical procedures that we have found helpful in our work with distressed marriages.

CHAPTER 1: GENERAL GUIDELINES AND PRINCIPLES

One of the major goals of the social learning approach to marital therapy is to increase the level of reciprocity between husband and wife. Reciprocity occurs when mutually pleasing or reinforcing exchanges and interactions punctuate the relationship. Of equal importance in promoting marital satisfaction is reducing the level of coercion in the relationship. Coercion occurs when partners get their needs and desires through threats, demands, and aversive control. Marital satisfaction is directly proportional to the frequency of mutually pleasing behaviors and inversely proportional to the frequency and intensity of mutual punishment. Anger, disappointment, frustration, and irritation are normal and expected feelings in a marriage; however, constructively dealing with these feelings makes the difference between successful and unsuccessful relationships.

The marital therapy espoused in this handbook is based on an educational model. Educating couples in positive ways to restructure their relationships means teaching new interactional skills. Learning new skills puts a focus on the present and the future; excessive dwelling on past unhappiness and problems is actively discouraged after an initial period of catharsis and evaluation. Serving as an educator, the therapist prompts, models, and coaches the couple in an active manner to bring about positive change in their behavior and attitudes. Practicing new skills in the safety of the clinic or office has to be followed by trying out the skills in the home and the real world. Therefore, homework is regularly assigned to help the couple use their newly learned skills in the natural environment.

CHAPTER 2: GETTING STARTED

An effective marital treatment approach is worth little unless adequate numbers of distressed married couples can be recruited and involved in the process. The therapist should make personal contacts with a variety of potential referral sources—clergy, physicians, probation officers, social welfare workers, community service clubs—and maintain a professional relationship with referring agents through systematic feedback that does not violate the patients' confidentiality.

The initial contact with a marital partner or couple is critical to subsequent therapeutic progress. There should be minimal waiting for the first appointment, and the married couple should receive a pleasant and positive impression from the start, avoiding feelings of being "just another case." The therapist can prevent or reduce ambiguities that lead to confusion by supplying specific information on fees, payment schedules, and expectations for the type of therapy.

A special problem in marital therapy occurs when only one spouse is willing to participate in therapy. Marital therapy with only one partner is possible but limited in its effects. It may be necessary for the therapist to work initially with the willing spouse toward the goal of involving the other partner; alternatively, the therapist may be able to persuade a reluctant spouse to attend one or several "evaluation" sessions by making a phone call directly. In the initial session, the therapist should make clear that assigning blame or guilt for problems is not helpful; that marital therapy does not mean that one or both partners are neurotic, crazy, or "sick"; and that it is understood that each partner is and will be trying to do the very best she or he can to improve the relationship. The therapist takes the role of the expert consultant to assist the couple in making changes in attitudes and actions that will improve the relationship.

While partners vary in their degree of commitment and motivation toward saving a marriage, it will be helpful for the therapist to insist that extramarital relations be taboo for the duration of therapy so that both spouses can invest all their time and energy in the change process. Temporary separation also hinders the therapeutic process, and the therapist may have to explain carefully why continuing to live together is important during therapy.

From the beginning, the therapist attempts to build a positive therapeutic alliance that is suffused with realistic expectations of outcome. Second honeymoons rarely last. The therapist should be sensitive to the balance and parity in the therapeutic relationship, especially if one spouse has had previous therapy, is more psychologically minded, or otherwise may be seen by the other to have an "advantage." Providing anecdotes about real couples and their problems and treatment can help to establish credibility and to cement the therapeutic relationship.

Early sessions are opportunities for ventilation and catharsis of feelings. Whether done in separate or joint sessions, the free expression of feeling and accumulated grievances is necessary for the couple to leave the past behind and to focus their attention and efforts on the present and the future. Together with appropriate marital inventories, questionnaires, and history taking, the free flow of stored-up emotions helps the therapist to evaluate the problems, strengths, and weaknesses of the marital dyad. Observing the interactions between the partners as they emerge in the first few sessions also provides clues to the problems and imbalances in the relationship. The therapist needs to be reminded to ask of the interaction patterns: "Who does most of the talking? Who does the listening? Who interrupts and tries to direct the topics? Who assigns blame and responsibility? Is there the potential for violence? What type of nonverbal communication occurs? Are there problems in physical closeness or contact?" Evaluation can also be aided by probing into the various arenas of marital interaction, such as money management, child management, recreation, sex, household management, and relations with friends, family, and other couples. Beyond evaluation, comprehensive clarification of these arenas of married life highlights who wants what from whom, similarities and differences in values and expectations, and hidden agendas and unconsciously held desires and demonstrates the importance of empathy, mutual tolerance, and tuning in to each other. Chapter 2 concludes with a practical checklist for starting marital therapy and with concrete suggestions on how to organize a marital therapy group.

CHAPTER 3: PLANNING RECREATIONAL AND LEISURE TIME

Many couples come for marriage counseling because of problems resulting from poor use of their time in social and recreational activities. Problems develop when too much or too little time is spent together, when overinvolvement with children or work occurs, when too much or too little time is spent with other couples and family. A mutually planned and well-balanced recreational and social life is necessary for the fire and life of a marriage relationship. Sometimes, all that is required to repair a torn marriage is teaching the couple how to better distribute and share their recreational and leisure time. Focusing on this arena of marriage early in therapy is also helpful because it directs the couple's attention away from tension and conflict toward fun and play, thereby injecting some positive feeling and optimism into a relationship previously burdened with despair.

The therapist can improve the recreational side of marriage by exploring a couple's time budget in four areas: (1) as individuals alone or with other people without the spouse's presence; (2) as a couple alone; (3) as part of a social group or with other couples; and (4) as a family with children and other relatives. While each spouse and couple have special and different needs in each of these areas, it is important to assist the couple to work toward agreement on how time is to be redistributed in the four areas. Doing this time budgeting in a marital group has definite advantages because of the exposure of each couple to a greater variety of alternatives, models, and preferences. When solitary recreation or time spent with a friend outside the dyad is viewed with concern, jealousy, or overdependence, the therapist may have to assist the threatened spouse with separate sessions or additional time for assertion training in developing his or her own abilities to satisfy recreational needs through hobbies or attachments to friends. Common complaints in marital therapy are "We don't have time to do things together like we used to do" or "We don't have enough money to go out anymore." While realistic time and financial limitations may exist, a creative searching for recreational opportunities often reveals a surprising number of interesting and promising possibilities for joint activities. The "Guide for Leisure-Time Planning," found in the

"Client's Workbook," can be filled out and be helpful in suggesting mutual choices and compromises.

CHAPTER 4: COMMUNICATING—AWARENESS OF RECIPROCITY

During our years of doing marital therapy, we have been consistently impressed with the overriding importance of training couples in communication skills. When spouses entering marriage counseling are polled on their biggest problem, they most frequently indicate poor communication. All arenas of marital life—sex, children, finances, household management, in-laws, friends, and recreation—are mediated by communication between the partners and their abilities to solve problems. We conceptualize the communication process as occurring in three steps: (1) accurately and sensitively recognizing incoming messages (receiving and listening skills); (2) being able to develop ideas or alternatives for responding to the situation, weighing the potential consequences of the possible alternatives, and choosing one that is reasonable (processing or cognitive skills); and (3) being able to respond with your own message, using effective verbal and nonverbal elements (sending skills). In Chapter 4, we discuss receiving skills; the processing and sending steps are described in Chapter 5.

Becoming more aware of the pleasing interactions and messages already occurring in a marriage is a useful starting point for a distressed couple. Not taking PLEASES for granted can be difficult for couples after years of routinized living together. To help sensitize spouses to the positive elements in each other, we offer exercises called "Reciprocity Awareness" and "Catch Your Spouse Doing or Saying Something Nice." Going through these exercises in the therapy sessions and at home raises each spouse's awareness and consciousness of things that make life easier and that make her or him feel better. The exercises also stimulate positive interaction and reinforce, through mutual acknowledgment, the already occurring satisfactions of the relationship.

CHAPTER 5: COMMUNICATING—THE ARTS OF LISTENING AND EFFECTIVELY EXPRESSING FEELINGS

Effective communication has two necessary components: a meaningful message and the ability to transmit that message. This chapter focuses on the training of content and style in marital relations and direct, congruent, empathic, and supportive communications. In the training procedure, the therapist coaches the clients in the nonverbal dimensions of communication, such as vocal volume, tone, facial expression, and eye contact.

A common problem encountered in marital therapy is the lack of listening skills. A tool used to enhance active listening skills is called the *executive session*, where the clients, in a safe, structured way, learn how to express, listen to, and provide feedback on progressively more complicated messages. The executive session helps a couple proceed in their communication of feelings stepwise from neutral to more sensitive topics. One partner expresses herself or himself without interruption by the other; then, the listener reflects or repeats back the essential content of the message to demonstrate that it has been understood; finally, the speaker provides feedback on the accuracy of the listener's reflection. The executive session format is used to practice various types of communication, such as asking for PLEASES, expressing negative feelings, and building empathy.

Perhaps the most difficult form of communication is the expression of negative and unpleasant feelings. We have found that harboring negative feelings invariably creates a tense and hostile relationship; the unpleasant emotions and attitudes have to come out in the open so that they can be dealt with constructively. These feelings are as much a part of a healthy relationship as positive emotions. We view sadness, hurt, annoyance, loneliness, and anger as feelings that should not be denied but dealt with. In expressing these feelings directly rather than beating about the bush, spouses are taught to own up to *their* feelings and to avoid accusing each other. Expression of hurt or angry feelings should take place not very long after the triggering event; gunnysacking, the accumulation of bad feelings, damages a positive relationship.

We consider empathy particularly crucial in intimate personal relations; thus it receives special attention in the training process. Skills are taught that are required to deal with unexpected hostility and persistent bad moods, including disarming with PLEASES, humor, changing the subject, time out, and ignoring.

We have found that many couples have problems exchanging physical affection and have to learn or relearn how to ask for a kiss, a hug, or sex verbally and nonverbally. Similarly, many partners have to realize the distinction between a request for physical affection and an overture to sexual relations. While sexual relations are not ignored in marital therapy, we do not provide, in this handbook, specific instructions on how to conduct sexual therapy. Some couples do just fine once they have established reliable signals, such as a particular dress; others need extensive training and homework assignments, while a third group needs referral for specific sexual treatment.

Spouses are taught to be assertive, not passive or aggressive. To promote positive problem-solving, the therapist should gain firsthand knowledge about the types of conflict that occur currently and regularly in the marriage. Rehearsing old resentments usually results in little payoff, while recent scrimmages are freshly in mind; thus, correct and incorrect ways of dealing with marital problems are meaningful. Role playing, rehearsal, and role reversal are vital techniques in acquiring the skill to express negative feelings in a positive manner. We suggest that the therapist play the complementary role, thus providing a safe setting for expression and observation. Instruction and coaching by the therapist will train the couple to handle stress situations at home. Videotape and audiotape feedback are often useful tools during office instruction. The techniques, tools, and instructions regarding effective listening and sending skills can be used in both dyadic and group settings.

CHAPTER 6: GIVING AND GETTING—MARITAL CONTRACTS

When the couple have learned to communicate effectively, they are ready for mutual agreements or contracts. In this manual, contracting is seen as a learning process in which the partners acquire the skills of specification, negotiation, and compromise. In this way, the couple gain a new tool to assist them in effective communication and in the management of conflict situations.

Contracting should be taught via a step-by-step approach in order to motivate practice and to assure success. The couple begin by making positive requests and slowly proceed to choosing responsibilities and privileges. The therapist will guide the couple so that the actions for negotiation are specifically defined regarding time, frequency, place, and circumstance. Several examples of faulty and correct ways of formulating items for negotiation are presented. Toward the end of Chapter 6, a sample contract is described, and a list of points to be used in reviewing an effective contract is offered.

Initially, the contracting procedure may be seen as artificial and contrived, but after some practice, the couple should acquire the basic skills and move to a more creative and spontaneous approach. The highly structured format may eventually be made more flexible, leaving the couple with a very effective tool that they can apply outside of the therapist's office.

CHAPTER 7: SOLVING SPECIAL PROBLEMS

Behaviorally oriented therapists are often criticized for assuming that the learning approach will be readily accepted by all clients. In fact, resistance to goals or to techniques is sometimes encountered. Chapter 7 offers the therapist several examples of methods for reaching that special, hard-to-deal-with couple.

A clear, matter-of-fact statement of goals by the therapist is often helpful in overcoming initial resistance and in creating reasonable expectations. The use of catharsis may set the stage for future positive work and may assist the therapist in identifying problem situations. Ventilation of feelings must be used with care, however, if effective communication and not catharsis is to be the goal of treatment. The therapist should also take time to listen to the couple's expectations in order to set attainable goals with which both the therapist and the couple can live. The therapist should also take time to listen to the couple's descriptions of any past experiences in therapy and to explain the comprehensive nature of the current therapy.

Some couples find the use of rehearsal and homework objectionable. The manual provides six possible ways of dealing with reluctance to participating in role playing. Resistance to homework can often be dealt with by more in-office practice to make the couple feel more secure in their attempts at home. If the assignments are "forgotten" because neither spouse takes the initiative, it may be necessary to have the spouses decide during the therapy session who is responsible for what. The recording forms should list specific, reasonable, and limited behaviors. Clients often report that the assignments feel mechanical. Therapist support and encouragement are crucial here to bridge the gap between initial success and acquiring proficiency, including spontaneity and creativity. The couple need to be reassured that, as with any other skill, lots of practice is needed before the behavior feels natural. The therapist is advised to give attention to the completed assignments and to ignore excuses for noncompletion.

Chapter 7 ends with various concrete suggestions for dealing with several problem situations that are not specific to the behavioral approach, including dropouts, outbursts and conflicts, and working with unwed couples. Careful screening, consistent ground rules, and developing backup resources are offered as effective means of preventive action.

CHAPTER 8: ENDING

As the therapy nears conclusion, problems thought to be resolved may recur, and behaviors assumed to have been mastered may mysteriously disappear. It is important to recognize these trends and to discuss them with the couple. Methods for dealing with the termination of therapy and avoiding problems include the use of time structure, fading procedures, the reinforcement of gains, the sharing of sadness, planning the future, and possible additional counseling.

Fading has been especially effective in averting termination problems. This can include scheduling sessions at longer intervals, a vacation from therapy, or offering one or more follow-up sessions. It may also be helpful if the couple plan to celebrate important dates and occasions in the future to increase togetherness and decrease apprehension. When a stress situation is foreseen, the therapist may plan for a brief visit by the couple to deal with that occasion.

Reviewing the gains made during therapy can be a powerful incentive in assisting the couple to continue on their own. The last session may be spent evaluating the various tools that the couple have acquired and discussing which techniques they have found effective and which they plan to continue to use in their regular interaction and in crisis situations. This procedure helps the couple to realize that they can use these tools on their own.

One of the last tasks in the therapeutic process is the completion of the "Marital Adjustment Test" and the "Client Satisfaction Questionnaire." These instruments are found in the "Client's Workbook."

CHAPTER 10: SUGGESTED SESSION OUTLINES FOR MARITAL THERAPY

Chapter 10 of the manual contains suggested outlines for 12 therapy sessions. While marital therapy should be personalized to fit the special needs of each couple, there is some advantage in having a semistandardized curriculum to guide the therapist through the comprehensive procedures described in the handbook. The session-by-session outlines for 12 therapeutic meetings, including a follow-up session, provide a point of departure for the therapist interested in using our recommended methods. These outlines will be particularly helpful to the novice therapist who has not had a large amount of experience working with married couples in distress.

CHAPTER 10

Suggested Session Outlines for Marital Therapy

Throughout this book, marital therapy has been viewed both as a problem-solving and an enrichment approach to marriages. We have offered suggestions and directions for conducting marital therapy in group settings as well as in the conjoint format with one couple alone. As it attempts to strengthen the unique relationship between partners in a wide diversity of couples, marital therapy has to remain flexible in the hands of the therapist or counselor. Therapists can become comfortable with our theoretical model and set of treatment techniques by incorporating these into their own personal and professional experiences and clinical style. Likewise, each couple should flexibly engage in the activities suggested in this manual, building on their unique histories as persons and as a couple. The variety and complexity of marital problems and growth possibilities make it necessary for the therapist to serve as a mediator and adaptor between this handbook and therapy. While we recognize the need to individualize and personalize the procedures of marital therapy, we would like to present in this chapter a therapist's guide, made up of outlines for a complete set of therapy sessions.

The session outlines serve as a curriculum for the therapist and may be particularly helpful to marriage counselors who are inexperienced and need structured guidance. As experience grows, departures can be made from the outlines to fit the special needs and interests of the therapist and the clients. This chapter, containing suggested procedures on a session-by-session basis, should not be read as a shortcut to the complete handbook, since many of the outlined procedures will make sense only against the background of what is described more fully in earlier chapters.

Few of the procedures listed have to take place in a particular session or sequence; however, we would strongly urge maintenance of the gradual approach within each problem area. For example, training of the communication skills should progress from neutral items to those with a greater emotional content. On the other hand, whether the couple's recreational activities are explored in the initial sessions or much later will depend on the personal preferences of the therapist and the needs and interests of each couple. Whereas one couple may need time to spend working on *core symbols* as a "safe" topic, another couple might be better off working on recreation to start off on a positive note. For others, the breakdown in communication may be so great that little can be accomplished until some basic interaction skills are learned or relearned.

These suggested guidelines may be of particular interest to you as a quick review and reminder of relevant interventions before starting a given session. One suggested format is to hold 7 weekly sessions, then 4 biweekly sessions, then a one-month follow-up session. We suggest that as the therapist, you make personal notes for each session and thereby create your own individualized outline. The text of the outline, with action-oriented information, is addressed to you, the therapist, unless otherwise indicated. It is up to you to present the necessary instructions in your own words and style to your patients.

SESSION 1

1. Welcome and overview of logistics, content, and format of marital therapy.
    a. Number and frequency of scheduled sessions.
    b. Fees.
    c. Communication with therapist between sessions.
2. Orientation.
    a. Confidentiality; specification of ground rules.
    b. Commitment to therapy.
        (1) Attendance at all sessions if at all possible.
        (2) Participation in exercises.
        (3) Completion of homework assignments.
        (4) Feedback on progress from therapist.
    c. In case of group marital therapy:
        (1) Each person introduces him/herself, starting with therapist as model.
        (2) Each person indicates why he/she is in therapy and what he/she hopes to accomplish.
3. Targeting of problems and goals.
    a. Ground rules for sessions.
    b. Focus on present and future, not the past.
    c. Problem definition in behavioral terms.

(1) Use positive goals.
(2) Explore alternatives.
(3) "What do you like about your spouse?"

4. Reciprocity in marriage.
   a. Dyad is the relevant marital unit.
   b. Each spouse has personal, social, emotional, and material needs.
   c. Giving and receiving PLEASES.
      (1) Theoretical explanation.
      (2) Hand out sample list of PLEASES.
      (3) Listing of PLEASES.
         (a) Currently received.
         (b) Currently given.
      (4) Practice giving and receiving PLEASES with couple.
      (5) Practice acknowledgement of PLEASES with couple.
5. Homework assignments for couple.
   a. List PLEASES currently being received or given (reciprocity awareness exercise).
   b. Record PLEASES (at least one a day) ("Catch Your Spouse Doing or Saying Something Nice").
   c. Acknowledge PLEASES.
   d. Perfect marriage procedure: Without consulting each other, spouses indicate what would make the marriage "perfect" with regard to one or more of the following: sex, communication, money, leisure time, social activities, household responsibilities, job, and independence/dependence.

SESSION 2

1. Reiterate ground rules.
   a. Confidentiality.
   b. Completion of homework assignments. Those who complete assignments will receive more of therapist's attention.
2. Review couple's homework.
   a. Review reciprocity awareness exercise.
   b. Review "Catch Your Spouse Doing Something Nice."
   c. Each spouse reads PLEASES received.
   d. Was acknowledgement given?
   e. Review perfect marriage procedure.

3. Practice giving and receiving PLEASES with couple.
    a. Therapist models appropriate behaviors.
    b. Be supportive of all attempts and approximations.
    c. Encourage mutual feedback.
4. Fantasy fulfillment procedure.
    a. Each spouse should list one new PLEASE that he/she would like from partner.
    b. Help spouses formulate new PLEASES.
    c. Spouses read lists of PLEASES aloud and negotiation is undertaken.
    d. Help spouses translate each desire into a continuum of possible activities.
5. Therapist or co-therapist demonstrates desirable and undesirable ways of asking for and giving physical affection.
    a. Explain importance of verbal and nonverbal communication of desires.
    b. Emphasize that change in behavior comes first, and change of feelings later.
6. Couple's homework assignments.
    a. Continue acknowledging PLEASES through the "Catch Your Spouse . . ." exercise.
    b. Each spouse is to carry out at least one mutually agreed-upon PLEASE.
    c. At least once a day, each spouse is to ask the other for some physical affection.

SESSION 3

1. Review homework with couple.
    a. Daily charting of PLEASES received using the "Catch Your Spouse . . ." exercise.
    b. Give positive feedback for spouses' efforts at acknowledging PLEASES.
    c. Review fantasy fulfillment exercise.
    d. Discuss the experiences of the couple in asking for physical pleasuring.
2. Further practice in fantasy fulfillment procedure with couple. In case of failure:
    a. Choose another, less sensitive area or topic.
    b. Scale down agreement to an easier task.
    c. Be specific in description of PLEASE.

    Therapist should use modeling and support all positive contributions from clients; role playing and behavior rehearsal are essential.

3. Core symbols: let each marriage partner describe examples of core symbols, that is, activities, events, places, or things that have special positive meaning in the marriage.
4. Evaluate progress made by the couple in their giving and acknowledging of everyday PLEASES. Have each partner demonstrate a PLEASE and have the other partner acknowledge it.
5. Practice communication skills with couple.
   a. Review essential value of reciprocity and communication in marriage.
   b. Practice expressing neutral statements.
   c. Practice listening skills: "I heard you say . . ."
   d. Practice expressing positive feelings.
   e. Use role reversal, modeling, feedback.
6. Homework assignments for couple.
   a. Continue "Catch Your Spouse . . ."
   b. Make list of core symbols (individually and/or as a couple).
   c. Offer daily practice (five minutes or more) of communicating and feedback of neutral and positive statements.

SESSION 4

1. Review couple's homework.
   a. Daily charting of PLEASES using the "Catch Your Spouse . . ." exercise.
   b. Core symbols—if couple has not brought a list, help them choose a core symbol in the session.
   c. Give experience in expressing neutral and positive statements, plus listening skills (What topics were used? How long did practice last?).
2. Practice communication skills with couple.
   a. Further practice of neutral and positive expressions.
   b. Teach the expression of negative feelings without hurting the other or being accusatory.
   c. Teach how to acknowledge negative feelings using empathy or shared meaning.
3. Therapist demonstrates various desirable and (in clearly exaggerated form) undesirable ways of expressing negative feelings. Therapist has one client express negative feelings in a desirable and an undesirable way and reacts accordingly.
4. Practice the expression of negative feelings, using modeling,

role reversal, behavioral rehearsal, and feedback. Emphasize both the verbal and the nonverbal components of communication skills.

5. Executive session.
   a. Explain the format.
   b. Conditions of place and time.
   c. Duration.
   d. Topic: for now, limited to neutral and positive items.
   e. Termination and feedback.
6. Couple's homework assignments.
   a. Continue "Catch Your Spouse . . ."
   b. Daily practice of expressing negative feelings, plus appropriate feedback.
   c. Begin executive sessions under conditions agreed upon during this session.

SESSION 5

1. Review of couple's homework.
   a. Daily charting of PLEASES.
   b. Experiences with expression of negative feelings.
   c. Executive sessions: neutral and positive topics.
      (1) Have couple repeat an executive session that was practiced at home.
      (2) Coach appropriate expression of feelings and further feedback.
      (3) Discuss problems in communication and do a rerun with more coaching to improve interaction.
2. Communication skills: negative feelings.
   a. Review guidelines.
   b. Demonstrate appropriate and inappropriate ways of expressing negative feelings.
   c. First separate and then combine verbal and nonverbal expressions.
3. Practice expression of negative feelings using the executive session format, and if possible, have each partner clearly exaggerate expressing negative feelings. In case of group therapy, allow for feedback by various group members, and have members take turns demonstrating their expression of negative feelings.

4. Recreation. In order to end on a positive note, have couple discuss their current and desired engagement in:
   a. Recreation as individuals.
   b. Recreation as a couple.
   c. Recreation as a couple with other couples.
   d. Recreation as a family.
5. Couple's homework assignments.
   a. "Catch Your Spouse . . ."
   b. Executive session: negative feelings.
   c. List recreational activities for each of the four categories delineated.

SESSION 6

1. Review of couple's homework.
   a. Daily charting of PLEASES.
   b. Forms and content of recreational activities.
   c. Communication skills (executive sessions): negative feelings.
2. Recreational activities.
   a. What areas are lacking for each individual spouse?
   b. For each couple alone?
   c. For each couple with other couples?
   d. As a family?

Determine at least one form of recreation that both partners enjoy either currently or potentially.

3. Communication skills.
   a. Review in detail problems being experienced by couple.
   b. Have couple replay an executive session practiced at home, especially if the session did *not* work out well.
   c. Discuss their efforts at conducting executive sessions, offer suggestions, and allow further practice.
4. Contingency contracting.
   a. Clarify and give rationale for the value of contracting.
   b. Emphasize the role of communication skills in contracting, especially the need for specificity and active listening.
   c. Stress the importance of reciprocity in contracting and how this strengthens a marriage.
   d. Distinguish between "bribes" and exchanging rewards through mutually acceptable compromises.

   e. Explain that the couple may initially feel contracting to be artificial but that this later disappears as the process becomes more spontaneous.
5. Contracting exercise.
   a. Introduce the "Family Happiness Index."
   b. Have each spouse choose a responsibility for himself or herself.
   c. Determine specifics of behavior.
   d. Spouses exchange responsibility cards and provide feedback.
   e. Spouses accept, reject, or negotiate a responsibility offered by partner.
6. Couple's homework assignments.
   a. Continue daily charting of PLEASES.
   b. Continue executive session on positive or neutral topics.
   c. Perform at least one mutually agreed-upon recreational activity as a couple.
   d. Carry out the negotiated responsibility from the contracting exercise.

SESSION 7

1. Review couple's homework.
   a. Spouses select and discuss three most appreciated PLEASES.
   b. Spouses report on executive sessions.
   c. Spouses report on recreational activities.
   d. Spouses report on compliance with negotiated responsibilities.
2. Communication skills: owning up to and directly expressing negative feelings. Each spouse is taught to express anger, hurt, irritation, frustration, fear, and helplessness in a direct way while the other spouse practices empathic listening, shared meaning, and reflecting back. The executive session format can be used.
3. Contracting exercise.
   a. Spouses review responsibilities chosen for themselves.
   b. Each spouse chooses a responsibility for his/her partner.
   c. Help spouses build empathy.
   d. Help spouses set costs on responsibilities.
4. Practicing contracting with couple.
   a. Accept the responsibility given by partner.

   b. Reject the responsibility.
   c. Negotiate and compromise until agreement and mutual satisfaction have been obtained.
   d. Coach the clients in communicating their desires while stressing the importance of listening to each other and of reciprocity.
5. Couple's homework assignments.
   a. Review and reiterate assignments of all sessions so far. Support positive reactions.
   b. Continue charting daily PLEASES through "Catch Your Spouse . . ." exercise.
   c. Continue practicing communication skills in executive sessions.
   d. Use one executive session for negotiating contract items.
   e. Carry out a negotiated responsibility.

SESSION 8

1. Review couple's homework.
   a. Ask each spouse to select most appreciated PLEASE received during past week.
   b. Report on executive session used for negotiating a contract.
   c. Discuss execution of negotiated responsibility.
2. Communication skills: additional instruction and practice based on a review of all previous sessions.
   a. Giving and acknowledging PLEASES.
   b. Expressing negative feelings.
   c. Reflecting back other's feelings: active listening skills.
   d. Executive sessions.
   e. Negotiating skills.
3. Communication skills: asking for PLEASES.
   a. Differentiate between affirmative/assertive requests for pleasing behavior and passive/aggressive ways of asking.
   b. Therapist models various behaviors and gives complete strategies for responding positively or negatively to requests for PLEASES.
   c. Couple practices asking for PLEASES.
   d. Couple practices saying no in a supportive, nonoffensive manner.
4. Communication skills: suggesting alternatives.
   a. Together with couple, explore various alternatives to a

given positive request. Brainstorming may be effective here.
   b. Model suggesting alternatives.
   c. Practice suggesting alternatives.
5. Review progress couple has made in recreation as a family.
6. Couple's homework assignments.
   a. Chart PLEASES received daily using the "Catch Your Spouse . . ." exercise.
   b. Practice communication skill of expressing negative feelings directly using the executive session format.
   c. Practice saying no to a positive request.
   d. Practice negotiating alternatives to a positive request and mutually choosing one or compromising for an agreement.

SESSION 9

1. Review couple's homework.
   a. Review on personal impact of PLEASES given and received.
   b. Review experiences that partners have had in expressing negative feelings in executive sessions.
   c. Give feedback to partners on their progress in saying no and generating alternatives to positive requests.
   d. Review progress in redistributing recreational and leisure time.
2. Check out with each spouse whether his or her inner, subjective feelings are beginning to correlate with his or her overt actions in noting, acknowledging, and giving PLEASES.
   a. Emphasize that each will get out of the therapy only what he/she puts into it.
   b. Do not belabor failure; be supportive.
   c. In case only one spouse seems actively involved:
      (1) Encourage the expression of negative feelings and help the partners share disappointments and irritation directly without accusations.
      (2) Point out positive changes; encourage patience.
3. Practice contingency contracting.
   a. Have each partner choose a privilege for herself or himself.
   b. Determine the specifics of the privilege.
   c. Have the partners exchange requests and have each accept the spouse's request if at all reasonable.
   d. Have each partner choose a privilege for the other.
   e. Get each partner to set values on the privileges chosen.

   f. Assist the couple in negotiating, bargaining, compromising, and agreeing.
4. Review the following communication skills:
   a. Acknowledging PLEASES.
   b. Initiating PLEASES.
   c. Giving feedback and making specific requests for physical affection.
   d. Expressing negative feelings.
   e. Using empathy.
   f. Assertively and positively asking for PLEASES.
5. Open-ended discussion on progress of therapy to date.
6. Couple's homework assignments.
   a. Continue daily charting of PLEASES.
   b. Carry out or make possible the privilege selected for spouse—and use one's own privilege.
   c. List unfulfilled expectations of therapy for review next session.
   d. Select and engage in one recreational activity for oneself, apart from the spouse.

SESSION 10

1. Review couple's homework.
   a. Review PLEASES given and received.
   b. Give feedback on privileges requested in contract.
   c. Report on recreation for self.
   d. List unfulfilled expectations.
2. Discussion of spouse's unfulfilled expectations.
   a. Specification of problems and goals.
   b. Communication of expectations.
   c. Long-range planning: importance of approximating expectations in small steps.
   d. End of therapy is approaching, so do not avoid or postpone conflicts or emotionally divisive issues.
3. Practice communication skills.
   a. Use executive session format to have each partner express his/her expectations for the future.
   b. Encourage the partners to listen to and accurately reflect back the unfulfilled expectations that each states, since these impressions may be crucial for the future.
4. Practice contingency contracting.
   a. Have couple negotiate expectations.

   b. Emphasize importance of patience, compromise, and support.
   c. Emphasize role of reciprocity.
5. Review progress and results achieved during therapy; have clients explain which skills learned in the therapy will be consolidated and used in the future.
6. Homework assignments.
   a. Continue to chart daily PLEASES.
   b. Couple should schedule an executive session to discuss unfulfilled expectations.

SESSION 11

1. Review couple's homework.
   a. Review of PLEASES given and received and how these can be exchanged more spontaneously in the future.
   b. Report on executive session dealing with unfulfilled expectations.
2. Practice communication skills.
   a. How to deal with unexpected displacement of hostility.
   b. How to deal with spouse's failure to comply with or fulfill a request or a promised action.
   c. How to cope with unexpected breakdowns in communication.
   d. How to cope with inexplicable bad moods, sulking, and withdrawal.
3. Focus on special needs of the couple, providing ample opportunity for them to use the therapist as a consultant.
4. Let each partner discuss his/her expectations at the start of therapy and the growth that the marriage has experienced.
5. Discuss termination.
   a. Encourage expressions of sadness, apprehension, and concern over ending.
   b. Help couple to formulate future goals.
   c. Solicit from each partner which coping skills learned in therapy will be practiced during the interval until the follow-up session.
   d. Referral to other agencies if this is required.
6. Couple's homework assignments.
   a. Encourage continuation of mutual exchange of PLEASES.
   b. Encourage use of executive sessions when problems arise.
   c. Self-selected assignments to be done before follow-up session.

FOLLOW-UP SESSION

1. Couple's homework.
   a. Review each spouse's self-selected assignment.
   b. Continue the use of PLEASES.
2. Each partner reports on progress made and difficulties experienced.
3. Therapist acts as consultant in problem solving and in reinforcing progress.
4. Offer problem-solving techniques for possible future conflicts and dissatisfactions.
5. Discuss resources available to couple in the community.

Annotated Bibliography of Research on Behavioral Approaches to Marital Therapy

As authors of the *Handbook of Marital Therapy*, we are aware of and sensitive to the ethical and professional hazards of offering a new technique for widespread and general use by marriage counselors, pastoral counselors, family therapists, and other mental health professionals and paraprofessionals. We would not recommend that others use the methods in our handbook unless the methods had been empirically evaluated and researched. The particular methods described in the handbook have received systematic scientific validation, both by ourselves and by other investigators using similar methods. In one study carried out by Liberman and his colleagues, a comparison between behavioral and interactional approaches to marital therapy in a community mental health center revealed that the married couples receiving the behavioral therapy displayed significantly more positive and mutually supportive verbal and nonverbal behaviors in their interactions as a result of treatment. This study was published as a monograph in *Acta Psychiatrica Scandinavica* in 1976 and is abstracted in this bibliography. Another evaluation of 40 spouses in five behaviorally led marital groups at the same community mental health center demonstrated an average rise in marital satisfaction of 12 points in the Locke–Wallace "Marital Adjustment Test," indicating that the group experience had a statistically significant as well as a clinically significant impact.

Despite the specificity and detail with which this book is written, we would encourage readers to avail themselves of additional training and supervision in behavioral therapy techniques and principles. Behavioral approaches to marital therapy are changing all the time in response to new research, and the busy clinician who is a neophyte in behavior therapy but who wishes to assimilate and put to use the material in this handbook would be well advised to obtain supervision by a professional with greater experience and competence in behavioral therapy.

Ten years of experimental research and program evaluations of the types of behavioral learning techniques included in this handbook have clearly demonstrated their effectiveness with married couples in distress. This body of research is summarized in this annotated bibliography. We have decided to provide readers of our handbook with a digest of the scientific research on behavioral approaches to marital therapy in bibliographic form rather than citing or reviewing the research in the text. In this manner, we hoped to avoid diluting the practical and clinical focus of the handbook.

ALEVIZOS, P. N., & LIBERMAN, R. P. Behavioral approaches to family crisis intervention. In H. L. P. Resnick & H. Parad (Eds.), *Innovations in emergency mental health services*. Bowie, Md.: Brady, 1975.

This chapter outlines the advantages of behavioral approaches to family crisis intervention. A behavioral formulation of crisis theory is proposed. The effects of reciprocal and coercive family interactions and patterns on crisis in the family are summarized. The procedures used in a behavioral approach to family crisis intervention are briefly presented and illustrated with three case examples.

AZRIN, N., NASTER, B. J., & JONES, R. Reciprocity counseling: A rapid learning-based procedure for marital counseling. *Behavior Research and Therapy*, 1973, *11*, 365–382.

The authors formulated a model of marital discord based on reinforcement theory, developed a marital counseling procedure based on that theory, and evaluated its effectiveness. The model views marital discord as the result of nonreciprocated reinforcement. The counseling procedures developed attempt to establish reciprocity of reinforcement between spouses by teaching positive exchanges in several areas of marital unhappiness. The reciprocity procedure was conducted for three to four weeks with 12 couples, after first conducting a catharsis type of counseling as a control procedure. Results showed that the reciprocity procedure increased reported marital happiness, whereas the control procedure did not.

Reciprocity counseling for specific problem areas generalized somewhat to other problem areas. Increases in marital happiness occurred for each of the specific problem areas of marital interaction for 96% of the clients and was maintained and increased during a one-year follow-up period.

BIRCHLER, G. R. & Spinks, S. Behavioral systems and family therapy: Integration and clinical application. *American Journal of Family Therapy*, 1980.

This article provides a preliminary theoretical integration of social learning theory and family systems theory. It also describes a therapeutic approach derived from this integration. Behavioral systems *conceptual* integration is exemplified by the authors' discussion of the development of family rules. The authors conclude that both systems and behavioral therapists often monitor similar behaviors and interpersonal processes. Furthermore, the main differences between the two approaches have consisted of (1) the language used to describe interactional phenomena, (2) the units of target behavior, and (3) the therapeutic procedures employed to bring about change. The article presents a rather detailed explication of the authors' multiple strategies for intervention, which are designed to integrate the major behavioral and family systems treatment techniques.

CROWE, M. *Evaluation of conjoint marital therapy.* Dissertation, 1976, University of Oxford, England.

Crowe randomly assigned 42 couples with marital problems and neurotic or sexual difficulties to one of three conjoint approaches. The first, a directive approach, was an operant-interpersonal or behavioral approach. The second was a group-analytic approach that used the interpretation of reported and observed interaction to induce unequivocal expression of feeling by the couple. The third approach utilized supportiveness, through which the therapist attempted to keep communication going but did not advise or interpret the interaction. Therapy sessions were tape-recorded and evaluated by raters blind to the procedures being utilized. Significant improvements were found for all three approaches on the "Marital Adjustment Scale"; on target problems that related to interactional or interpersonal problems; and on those target problems that related to personal or psychiatric problems. However, the behavioral approach showed significantly greater improvement on these indices compared with the other two approaches and was also the only treatment to show a statistically significant improvement between pre- and post-treatment ratings on the "Sexual Adjustment Scale."

EISLER, R. M., HERSEN, M., & AGRAS, W. S. Effects of videotape and instructional feedback on nonverbal marital interaction: An analog study. *Behavior Therapy,* 1973, 4(4), 551–558.

The separate and combined effects of videotape feedback and focused instructions were examined in an analog study of 12 couples' marital interaction. Results indicated that videotape feedback in the absence of instructions effected a slight increase in nonverbal interactions of the couples. Focused instructions led to marked changes in the target behaviors. The combination of videotape feedback and focused instructions did not appear superior to focused instructions alone.

Greer, S. E., & D'Zurilla, T. J. Behavioral approaches to marital discord and conflict. *Journal of Marriage and Family Counseling*, 1975, *1*, 299–315.

This article is a review of the empirical research in behavioral approaches to marital therapy. The level and rigor of current research designs were evaluated as not having yet advanced beyond the nonfactorial single-group design, and the breadth of treatment populations employed thus far has been restricted. The power of the behavioral method was found in its theoretical base, its use of observational and treatment-relevant assessment, its procedural specificity, and its quantification of outcome. The outcomes of treatment, though relatively small in number thus far, have been almost universally positive and encouraging.

Gurman, A. S. The effects and effectiveness of marital therapy: A review of outcome research. *Family Process*, 1973, *12*(2), 145–170.

The literature on outcome research in marital therapy was reviewed. The issues considered included the nature of outcome criteria, the need to establish a baseline against which to measure improvement, and therapeutic effectiveness as a function of treatment type and time in therapy. The overall improvement rate across a heterogeneous collection of patients, therapists, and treatment modalities was 66%. This finding suggested, conservatively, at least a moderately positive therapeutic effect in light of the judgment that spontaneous rates of improvement appear to be much lower in marital than in individual therapy. Evidence of deterioration in couples undergoing marital therapy was also discovered.

Gurman, A. S., & Kniskern, D. P. Research on marital and family therapy: Progress, perspective and prospect. In S. L. Garfield & A. E. Bergin (Eds.), *Handbook of psychotherapy and behavior change: An empirical analysis* (2d ed.). New York: Wiley, 1978.

This excellent review article traces the history of marital and family therapy and critically examines studies of both behavioral and nonbehavioral marital and family therapy. While all forms of marital therapy appear to bring about favorable changes in couples, the behavioral approaches have been evaluated with a wider range of outcome measures and show a somewhat stronger impact on distressed marriages.

An analysis of factors influencing therapy outcome for selected clinical populations is provided based on trends emerging from their comprehensive analysis. Marriage enrichment programs and divorce therapy are discussed. The authors have also considered evidence of deterioration from such treatment. Recommendations for further study are offered, and the implications for training and practice of marital and family therapy are considered from a clinical perspective. Although some of the subject matter for this review concerns family therapy, the authors focused their concern on whether treatment and the resultant outcome alters the interaction between or among family members. This *relationship* focus provides generalizable implications for marital therapy.

HOPS, H., WILLS, T., WEISS, R., & PATTERSON, G. Marital interaction coding system. Unpublished manuscript, 1971. Copies may be obtained by writing to Dr. R. Weiss, Psychology Clinic, Department of Psychology, University of Oregon, Eugene, Ore. 97403.

The Marital Interaction Coding System (MICS) is used to objectively record verbal and nonverbal negotiations of marital problems between marriage partners. Codings of behaviors exhibited by the couple that can be classified using 28 well-defined verbal and nonverbal categories are made sequentially in 30-second blocks by trained coders. Extensive use of the MICS in recording the interactions of married couples demonstrates that these 28 categories are sufficient to provide an adequate accounting of the behavior that takes place in a problem-solving session. This manuscript is a manual describing and illustrating the use of the MICS. The 28 behavioral categories are defined, and the training procedures for coders using the MICS are given.

JACOBSON, N. Marital problems. In R. P. Liberman (Ed.), *Symposium on Behavior Therapy in Psychiatry, Psychiatric Clinics of North America*, Vol. 1, No. 2. Philadelphia: Saunders, 1978.

In this chapter, the author described the primary treatment strategies derived from a behavioral exchange model of relationship distress and outlined the theoretical assumptions that serve as the basis for these treatment strategies. The behavioral model of marital distress assumes that the amount of "pleasing" behavior that partners direct toward their mates, as well as their degree of subjective satisfaction with the relationship, is largely a function of how the mates respond. Much as communication theorists, behaviorists view the marital relationship as a system, where each partner's behavior is being maintained by reinforcement from the other.

The basic treatment strategies based on these assumptions and accumulated evidence are described and illustrated. These strategies include teaching couples behavior change skills, communication skills, problem-solving skills, and contracting skills. Additional focuses include rectifying sexual problems and training couples to maximally increase their positive behaviors in the relationship by identifying important rewards and punishments for their spouses. The author has also provided an overview of the studies that empirically support behavioral types of marital therapy.

JACOBSON, N., & WEISS, R. L. Behavioral marriage therapy: III. The contents of Gurman et al. may be hazardous to our health. *Family Process,* 1978, *17,* 149–163.

This paper was written as a reply to a critique of behavioral marital therapy (BMT) by Gurman, Kniskern, and Knudson.[1] The reply is divided into four sections. First, the paper addresses the critics' comments on the conceptual model put forth by BMT, correcting and clarifying various misconceptions, presented as fact by Gurman *et al.,* and restating some of the basic ideological principles in the behavioral model. Second, the paper discusses behavioral change techniques and technology, along with extratechnological treatment considerations. Again, misrepresentations of BMT are corrected. Third, an analysis of the literature investigating the therapeutic efficacy of BMT is reviewed, and the conclusion is reached that BMT is demonstrably effective, at least for a substantial number of mildly to moderately distressed couples. Criticisms are made of the analysis of the same literature conducted by Gurman *et al.* The authors have concluded that contrary to the spirit of the papers by Gurman *et al.,* BMT is a viable framework for conceptualizing and treating relationship problems and that the commitment of its adherents to experimental investigation promises continued evolution, refinement, and improvement.

JACOBSON, N. S. Problem solving and contingency contracting in the treatment of marital discord. *Journal of Consulting and Clinical Psychology,* 1977, *45,* 92–100.

Ten married couples reporting dissatisfaction with their relationship were randomly assigned to an experimental treatment group and to a

[1]A. S. GURMAN, & R. M. KNUDSON, Behavioral marriage therapy: I. Psychodynamic-systems analysis and critique, *Family Process,* 1978, *17,* 121–138; and A. S. GURMAN, & D. P. KNISKERN, Behavioral marriage therapy: II. Empirical perspective. *Family Process,* 1978, *17,* 139–148.

minimal treatment waiting-list control group. Couples in the experimental group were trained to interact more positively through the process of trial and error. Therapists interrupted couples' inappropriate problem-solving behavior, explained what was wrong with their response, suggested an appropriate alternative, and modeled and role-played these alternatives. Couples also engaged in supervised practice of appropriate problem-solving behavior, were taught to negotiate contracts, and completed homework assignments between sessions.

Pre- and postobservational measures of the couples' interactions indicated significant changes in the desired directions: positive interactions increased and negative interactions decreased. No changes in interaction were observed in the control group. Mean scores on the self-report index of marital satisfaction, the "Marital Adjustment Scale," indicated increased marital satisfaction from pre- to posttest in the experimental group and no change in the control group. These changes were maintained in the experimental group as of one year following treatment.

JACOBSON, N. S. Specific and nonspecific factors in the effectiveness of a behavioral approach to the treatment of marital discord. *Journal of Consulting and Clinical Psychology*, 1978, *46*, 442–452. (a)

This study compared two behavioral treatments for marital discord with a nonspecific control and a waiting-list control. The behavioral treatments combined training in problem-solving skills with training in contingency management procedures, differing only with respect to the contracting form: one group learned to form good-faith contracts, and the other, *quid pro quo* contracts. Thirty-two couples were randomly assigned to one of these treatment conditions and one of three therapists. Improvement was assessed by two observational measures and by two self-report questionnaires. On all measures, both behavioral groups improved significantly more than waiting-list couples. On three of the four measures, behavioral couples improved significantly more than nonspecific couples. The two behavioral groups did not differ from one another on any of the measures.

JACOBSON, N. S. A stimulus control model of change in behavioral couples' therapy: Implications for contingency contracting. *Journal of Marriage and Family Counseling*, 1978, *4*, 35–39. (b)

Although contingency contracting is a popular strategy for use in treating distressed relationships, there is no direct evidence of its efficacy. A stimulus control model of change in behavioral therapy with couples states that the conditions under which an agreement was negotiated, regardless of the consequences specified in the agreement itself, are the primary determinants of whether the agreement is upheld. Once change is prompted, its maintenance is associated with stimuli generated by the negotiating session itself (that is, self-statements) and contingencies provided by concurrent changes occurring in therapy. Therefore, it is argued that explicit contingency contracting is unnecessary and may be contraindicated in cases where couples are distrustful and feeling manipulated by the spouse. Hypotheses are offered that provide indirect tests of this model of change in behavioral therapy for couples.

JACOBSON, N. S. Behavioral treatments for marital discord: A critical approach. In M. Hersen, R. M. Eisler, & P. M. Miller (Eds.), *Progress in behavior modification*. New York: Academic, 1979. (a)

This review of behavioral approaches to marital discord examines the theory, measurement, and treatment approaches developed in this area during the past 10 years. The major theoretical view of behavior therapists has been that marital discord is a function of a low rate of positive reinforcers exchanged between spouses. Four separate measurement strategies have produced a convergence of findings that are consistent with the view that distressed couples exhibit fewer rewarding and more punishing interactions than nondistressed couples. Research has accumulated on the development of disturbed marital interaction with the following important determinants: (1) deficits in behavior change and/or problem-solving skills; (2) the gradual loss of the reinforcing value of a spouse's behavior over time because of satiation or habituation; and (3) individual differences between the two spouses in their tendency to rely on interpersonal intimacy, as opposed to independent activities.

Self-report instruments, spouse-observation instruments, and behavioral ratings by trained observers each have their own use and function in the measurement of marital distress. Behavioral therapy approaches for marital discord derive from two major themes. One emphasizes behavioral exchange and results in therapy sessions structured to facilitate the negotiated exchange of positive behaviors, frequently with a contingency contract as a product. The second theme emphasizes teaching couples communication and problem-solving skills. The results of outcome studies on behavioral marital therapy suggest that approaches or therapeutic packages that combine training in problem-solving skills with contingency contracting and other behavioral exchange methods are effective.

JACOBSON, N. S. A review of the research on the effectiveness of marital therapy. In T. J. Paolino, Jr., & B. S. McCrady (Eds.), *Marriage and marital therapy: Psychoanalytic, behavioral, and systems theory perspectives.* New York: Brunner/Mazel, 1979. (b)

This chapter is organized into subsections, each of which reviews important experiments within a particular area of outcome investigations in marital therapy. The first section, on methodology, defines the characteristics and domain of outcome research. The authors have provided summaries of the two areas of marital therapy about which a substantial body of outcome literature has accumulated: communication training and contingency management. An overview of studies on a variety of approaches relevant to the treatment of couples concludes with a summary of studies that have successfully applied behavioral marital therapy to two clinical problems: alcoholism and sexual dysfunctions.

JACOBSON, N. S., & MARTIN, B. Behavioral marriage therapy: Current status. *Psychological Bulletin,* 1976, *83*(4), 540–556.

The literature on behavioral approaches to marriage therapy is reviewed. First, theories regarding the nature, etiology, and maintenance of marital problems are presented; second, behavioral approaches to treatment are described; and third, attempts to assess the efficacy of these treatments are evaluated. Although there is some highly suggestive evidence that behavioral interventions are effective, conclusive demonstrations have not been forthcoming. But, as the authors also point out, no traditional therapeutic approach to marriage counseling has received direct empirical support in the literature, and the growth and application of social learning principles to marriage counseling may signal a new era of progress in marital therapy. On the basis of the literature, a number of suggestions are made for further research, including better controls over potentially relevant variables; investigations of the relative effectiveness of therapeutic components; and utilization of better outcome criteria, including multiple measures and direct observation of behavioral changes.

LIBERMAN, R. Behavioral methods in group and family therapy. *Seminars in Psychiatry,* 1972, *4*, 145–156.

This article provides a comprehensive picture of the variety of methods used by behavior therapists in therapy groups and in working with couples and families. The author has described the use of behavioral methods in (1) nondirective group therapy, in which there is no interference with spontaneous group interaction, and (2) directive group therapy, in which the therapy format is structured according to the nature of the behavioral problem or the method being applied. In this situation, the therapist takes a more task-oriented educational role with the group. This approach is discussed with regard to group desensitization programs and assertiveness-training groups.

The author has also addressed the ways that behavior modification is used in family therapy and illustrates this approach with a case example. The author has concluded that the behavioral approach to group and family therapy makes it less likely that a therapist will reinforce or model contradictory behavior patterns and that the behavioral approach is an efficient and effective means of modifying behavior regarding family and group systems.

LIBERMAN, R. P. Behavioral approaches to family and couple therapy. *American Journal of Orthopsychiatry,* 1970, *40,* 106–118.

This article describes how positive and negative family interactions can be understood in terms of the contingencies that reward maladaptive behavior. In order for positive changes to occur, family members must learn to give each other recognition and approval for desired behaviors. The therapist's task is to collaborate with the family or couple to (1) specify the maladaptive behaviors; (2) choose reasonable goals that are alternative, adaptive behaviors; and (3) direct and guide the family to change the contingencies of their social reinforcement patterns for maladaptive to adaptive target behaviors. Liberman also discusses three technical concerns for therapists working with families. These concerns are (1) creating and maintaining a positive therapeutic alliance; (2) making a behavioral analysis of the problem(s); and (3) implementing the behavioral principles of reinforcement and modeling in the context of ongoing interpersonal interactions. Four case examples are presented to illustrate the application of these behavioral approaches. The discussion section compares and contrasts behaviorally oriented and psychoanalytic family therapy.

LIBERMAN, R. P., KING, L. W., DERISI, W. J., & MCCANN, M. *Personal effectiveness: Guiding people to assert themselves and improve their social skills.* Champaign, Ill.: Research Press, 1975.

This guide is intended for professionals who desire a step-by-step or a how-to-do-it manual for working with individuals needing enlargement and refinement of their social and emotional skills. The procedures described in *Personal Effectiveness* are the cornerstone of the training of communication skills in marital therapy described in Chapter 5 of the *Handbook of Marital Therapy*. Personal-effectiveness training procedures include: goal setting, behavioral rehearsal, modeling, prompting, instructions, shaping, positive feedback, outside-of-clinic assignments, and reporting back to the therapist. This guide, together with the accompanying "Program Guide" for trainers, "Client's Introduction" brochure, and demonstration film can be used to learn these therapy procedures.

Liberman, R. P., Levine, J., Wheeler, E., Sanders, N., & Wallace, C. J. Marital therapy in groups: A comparative evaluation of behavioral and interactional formats. *Acta Psychiatrica Scandinavica*, Supplement 266, 1976.

A comparative evaluation was conducted in a community mental health center between two types of brief, marital therapy in groups. The four couples in the behavioral group received training in three areas: specifying and acknowledging how each spouse could please the other in reciprocal ways; engaging in behavioral rehearsals to learn more constructive verbal and nonverbal communication; and negotiating an agreement with the contingency contract. Therapists helped the five couples in the interactional group by establishing cohesiveness through encouraging group members to ventilate feelings and share similar problems; by promoting empathy, warmth and concern; by encouraging group members to describe problems and dissatisfactions more specifically and clearly without blaming; by suggesting ways that the couples could improve their relationship; and by giving feedback to provide group members with insight and awareness into their interpersonal behavior.

Outcome measures showed few differences between the groups on a variety of self-report measures; however, there were significant improvements by both groups on these measures after therapy and at the six-month follow-up evaluation point. The direct observation data indicated that the couples in the behavioral group displayed significantly more positive and mutually supportive verbal and nonverbal behaviors in their interaction as a result of treatment.

Liberman, R. P., & Roberts, J. Contingency management of neurotic depression and marital disharmony. In H. Eysenck (Ed.), *Case studies in behavior therapy*. London: Routledge & Kegan Paul Ltd., 1975.

This case study reports on the use of a variety of behavioral methods used by a community mental health center with a 30-year-old woman with neurotic depression. The woman participated in the credit incentive system of the center's day treatment program to increase her participation in constructive activities, to improve her grooming, to increase her rate of conversation, and to decrease her verbalizations about feeling sick and worthless. After one month of treatment, positive changes in each of these areas had occurred. Marital therapy with the woman and her husband was started because it was felt by the staff that unless her marital interactions changed for the better, she would continue to be susceptible to depression.

The woman and her husband had a very distant relationship and spoke very little to each other. It was felt that the couple's withdrawal from each other produced a critical loss of social reinforcers for the woman, which led to her depression.

The main part of the marital therapy consisted of the couple's exchanging or contracting for desired behaviors from each other. A contingency contract was drawn up in which the woman would dress more modishly and show more affection to her husband (which her husband wanted) and the husband would spend less time on his job and more at home and less time in private reading. The couple gave each other written receipts when the contract was fulfilled by one or the other.

The couple indicated a renewed willingness to continue the marriage and to work for further improvements. Sexual intercourse was resumed, and the couple reported greater satisfaction for the first time in five years.

A transcript of a follow-up interview three years after treatment ended is included.

LIBERMAN, R. P., WHEELER, E., & SANDERS, N. Behavioral therapy for marital disharmony: An educational approach. *Journal of Marriage and Family Counseling*, 1976 (October), 383–395.

After a description of the therapeutic assumptions behind a behaviorally based married couples group, initial intake, screening, and orientation procedures are discussed. The main therapeutic elements of this approach to marital treatment are described and illustrated with case examples. These elements are pinpointing and discriminating PLEASES; increasing the recognition, initiation, and acknowledgement of pleasing interactions; using core symbols to bring back warm, positive memories; redistributing the time spent in recreational and social activities; training the couple in communication skills following the format outlined in *Personal Effectiveness* (Liberman, King, DeRisi, & McCann, 1975) initiating pleasing behavior; acknowledging pleasing behavior;

assertiveness training; communicating negative feelings; verbal and nonverbal sexual communications; contingency contracting; and using executive sessions (preplanned and structured conversations during which the couple practice expressing their feelings to each other). These treatment elements are offered during 8–10 sessions spaced over a three-month period. The specific techniques are imbedded in a matrix consisting of group cohesiveness and an alliance between the spouses and the co-therapists.

Cumulative results from five groups (40 spouses) using this format indicated significant gains following treatment on the Locke–Wallace "Marital Adjustment Test." Couples' responses to the "Areas of Change Questionnaire" also showed improvement, with the spouses indicating significantly less desire for change in their partners after treatment.

LOCKE, H. J., & WALLACE, K. M. Short marital-adjustment and prediction tests: Their reliability and validity. *Marriage and Family Living*, 1959 (August), 251–255.

The best items or predictors from previous tests used to test or predict marital adjustment were selected to construct this instrument, which was then tested for reliability and validity on a new sample. This testing resulted in the selection of 15 items for the adjustment test and 35 for the predictor test. The Locke–Wallace "Marital Adjustment Test" has been used in a large number of studies of marriage counseling for screening and as a dependent measure of outcome or change. It is considered a standard instrument that can discriminate satisfied marriage partners from those who are distressed in their marriages. Because of its validity, sensitivity to change, and widespread use, the authors of the *Handbook of Marital Therapy* have included it as a means for determining the effectiveness of marital treatment. Copies of the "Marital Adjustment Test" are included in the "Client's Workbook" for this purpose.

MARGOLIN, G. A comparison of marital interventions: Behavioral, behavioral-cognitive, and nondirective. Paper presented at the Western Psychological Association Convention, Los Angeles, 1976.

Margolin compared three types of interventions for distressed marriages. A behavioral approach was designed to accelerate the rate of exchange of desirable relationship behaviors and to increase each partner's power to mediate rewards for the other. A behavioral–cognitive approach was built on the basic behavioral model but expanded with the addition of cognitive restructuring to negate the destructive feelings that one spouse held for the other and to define all outcomes in terms of mutual gains. A nondirective approach focused on the expression, reflection, and clarification of each spouse's feelings and relationship expectations. Twenty-seven couples were randomly assigned to one of the three treatment groups. The behavioral–cognitive approach was significantly superior to the other two approaches according to the couples' self-report of satisfaction on the Locke–Wallace "Marital Adjustment Test." Couples in both behavioral groups, compared with the nondirective group, exchanged significantly more pleasing events according to pre- and postobservational data recorded by each spouse at home. Analysis of videotaped samples of each couple's problem-solving behavior revealed that couples in both behavioral treatments displayed more of these behaviors at posttreatment testing than did nondirective couples. However, the behavioral–cognitive treatment was significantly superior to the behavioral treatment in this regard.

MARGOLIN, G. A multilevel approach to the assessment of communication positiveness in distressed couples. *International Journal of Family Counseling*, 1978, *6*, 81–89.

This study examines the association between several measures used to assess positive communications and communication skillfulness in distressed marital couples. A correlational matrix was used to present three observer sources (husband, wife, and trained other) crossed with three observational targets (husband's communication positiveness, wife's communication positiveness, and relationship adjustment). Significant correlations were found among all pairs of observers for marital adjustment scores but not for communication behaviors. All observers perceived a high degree of reciprocity between spouses in their outputs of positive communications, but positive communication behaviors did not correlate with marital satisfaction. The data suggest that caution must be exercised in making interpretations on the basis of single assessment procedures, particularly spouses' observations of self and partner. This research and that of others suggest that the exchange of negative communications may be a better predictor and correlate of marital satisfaction than the exchange of positive feelings and events.

MARGOLIN, G., & WEISS, R. L. Communication training and assessment: A case of behavioral marital enrichment. *Behavior Therapy*, 1978, *9*, 508–520.

A technology is presented for training marital partners in self-defined communication skills, and a method is described for assessing change across three observational sources (self, spouse, and trained others). By use of cueing and feedback procedures, spouses' skills in emitting helpful communication responses are enhanced and their mutual identification of such helpful responses is increased. The program included training to increase the couples' at-home exchange of pleasurable relationship events and training in contracting skills. Case study data are presented that reflect the necessity for multidimensional assessment. Results indicated an increase in communication, helpful responses, and spouse agreement that helpful responses had occurred. An increase in problem-solving skills was observed by trained coders, thereby establishing greater generality of the effect.

OLSON, D. H. Marital and family therapy: Integrative review and critique. *Journal of Marriage and the Family*, 1970, *32*, 501–538.

Olson has surveyed the emerging fields of marital and family therapy in terms of their developments in research, theory, and clinical practice. A system analysis was developed for categorizing the various clinical approaches in marital and family therapy. Several ways of bridging the professional gap between therapists and researchers are suggested. Recommendations for interdisciplinary borrowing are indicated, and exemplary projects giving new direction to the fields are discussed.

OLSON, D. H. Review and critique of behavior modification research with couples and families: Or are frequency counts all that really counts? Paper presented at the annual meeting of the Association for the Advancement of Behavior Therapy, New York, 1972.

This paper reviews and critiques various studies that evaluate the effectiveness of behavior therapy treatment programs with couples and families. A system analysis approach is presented to evaluate and review these studies, and methodological and conceptual limitations are described. The five system levels of marital and family treatment outcome measurement identified by Olson are (1) intrapersonal; (2) interpersonal; (3) quasi-interactional; (4) interactional; and (5) transactional. Studies utilizing measures that tap each of these outcome areas are discussed. Most of the studies reviewed were found to have measures at only one or two of the five system levels. Rationale and techniques are presented for increasing the scope and validity of these studies by including concepts and measures from the other system levels.

PATTERSON, G. R., HOPS, H., & WEISS, R. A social learning approach to reducing rates of marital conflict. Paper presented at the annual meeting of the Association for the Advancement of Behavior Therapy, New York, 1972.

This report outlines a preliminary stage in the development of a set of clinical techniques for behavioral marital therapy and their accompanying assessment procedures. The procedures were designed to alleviate marital conflicts in moderately distressed couples. Major intervention goals included the acquisition by the couple of the problem-solving skills necessary to constructively negotiate changes in each other's behavior; reduction of the levels of aversive stimuli exchanges; and an increase in the level of positive reinforcers. The general therapy techniques employed modeling, role playing, and videotape feedback of the couples' interaction. Observational data obtained using the Marital Interaction Coding System (MICS) showed a substantial number of significant changes in the expected direction for both husbands and wives. The self-report data for reported rates of pleasures and displeasures received from their spouses also showed statistically significant changes in positive directions for all but one of the comparisons.

PATTERSON, G. R., HOPS, H., & WEISS, R. Interpersonal skills training for couples in early stages of conflict. *Journal of Marriage and Family Counseling*, 1975, *37*, 295–303.

Videotape was used to teach 10 couples nonaversive labels and to be behaviorally specific when requesting changes of their spouses. Couples were taught to listen without reacting aversively and to negotiate conflicts according to the *quid pro quo* interchange format. Couples were also encouraged to engage in love days, in which one spouse trebled the number of reinforcers given the other. Analysis of pretherapy, during-therapy, and posttherapy videotaped interactions indicated significant increases in facilitating behaviors for both husbands and wives. If changes occurred in one member, changes occurred in the other. Disruptive behaviors decreased. Self-report measures indicated significant increases in the number of PLEASES received by each spouse. However, the rate of DISPLEASES decreased for the husbands but not for the wives.

RAPPAPORT, A. J., & HARRELL, J. A behavioral-exchange model for marital counseling. *The Family Coordinator*, 1972, *21*, 203–212.

An approach to marriage counseling based on the principles of reciprocity and social exchange is described. Behavior modification techniques are utilized to implement this program, which is designed to resolve marital conflict between spouses. Following an educational model throughout the program, spouses are encouraged to negotiate their own reciprocal-exchange contracts with decreasing dependency on the counselor–educator. A case study is presented to illustrate the functional utility of the model.

STUART, R. B. Operant-interpersonal treatment for marital discord. *Journal of Consulting and Clinical Psychology*, 1969, *33*(6), 675–682.

The behavioral approach to marital therapy described in this article is based on the assumption that successful and unsuccessful marriages can be differentiated by their adequacy in providing reciprocal positive reinforcements for each partner. Following the clarification of behavioral change objectives for both partners, Stuart has described a four-step treatment approach that culminates in the increased exchange of positive responses on a reciprocal basis. Data from four couples are presented, illustrating increases in the average daily hours of conversation and weekly rate of sex. Couples' self-report of marital satisfaction on an assessment inventory indicated that the rate of reported satisfaction increased in association with the reported behavioral changes. Couples' satisfaction inventory scores showed further increases for three of the four couples 24 weeks after treatment ended.

WEISS, R. L., HOPS, H., & PATTERSON, G. R. A framework for conceptualizing marital conflict: A technology for altering it, some data for evaluating it. In L. A. Hamerlynck, L. D. Handy, & E. J. Mash (Eds.), *Behavior change: Methodology, concepts, and practice*. Champaign, Ill.: Research Press, 1973.

This chapter summarizes an assessment and intervention package developed for couples experiencing marital conflict. This approach explicitly trains married couples in the use of behavior change principles, such as shaping, use of positive (not aversive) control, pinpointing, and contingency management. These techniques are combined with specific training in problem-solving behaviors and in the exchange of reinforcing behaviors with one another. The self-report and observational techniques used by the authors are briefly described and are illustrated with examples and data from couples in their program. Data from two studies evaluating the overall effectiveness of the treatment package are presented. Results of these studies indicated that the package is effective in producing the kinds of postintervention change one would deem important.

WEISS, R. L., BIRCHLER, G. R., & VINCENT, J. P. Contractual models for negotiation training in marital dyads. *Journal of Marriage and the Family,* 1974 (May), 321–330.

This paper describes the similarities and differences in contracting and negotiation procedures used in the "outside world" and in the marital dyad. Two major categories of contracting were developed within a behavioral framework. The *quid pro quo* contractual exchange model provides the greatest contingency control; however, there are numerous difficulties associated with its use in marital dyads. The implicit-exchange, or good-faith, contractual format seems to fit more easily into the overall goals of marital therapy. The authors have illustrated uses of each of these contractual models in marital counseling and have noted each of their strengths and weaknesses.

WILLIAMS, A. M. The quantity and quality of marital interaction related to marital satisfaction: A behavioral analysis. Doctoral dissertation, University of Florida, Gainsville, 1977.

Ten "happily married" couples and ten distressed couples in marital therapy were compared on the quantity and quality of time spent in husband–wife interaction. Each spouse recorded the amount and perceived quality of time spent with the other for 14 consecutive days. The two groups were significantly different in the end-of-day ratings of marital happiness of both husband and wife. Highly significant differences were also found between the two groups in husband–wife *agreement* on rating of the *quality* of ongoing marital interaction, although there were no significant differences in agreement between husband and wife on the *quantity* of time they had spent together. Interaction patterns monitored included pleasant, neutral, and unpleasant behaviors, as well as daily and weekly interaction schedules and sequences. Simultaneous husband–wife monitoring of the duration, content, and quality of daily interaction sequences is proposed as a useful evaluative procedure for identifying the behavioral strengths and deficiencies of a particular marital relationship.

WILLS, T. A., WEISS, R. L., & PATTERSON, G. R. A behavioral analysis of the determinants of marital satisfaction. *Journal of Consulting and Clinical Psychology,* 1974, *42*(6), 802–811.

Seven couples with stable marriages made daily observations of spouses' pleasurable and displeasurable behavior for 14 consecutive days. They also made daily ratings of the enjoyability of their outside experiences (not with spouse) and of their satisfaction with the relationship. Couples' self-report of their satisfaction with the quality of their marital interaction was used as a criterion variable to assess the relative contribution of pleasurable and displeasurable events. Instrumental (meals and shopping, child care, finances, etc.), and affectional behaviors were positively related to marital satisfaction, whereas displeasurable behaviors were negatively related to satisfaction.

The article that follows was published after the handbook was typeset. Since it is relevant to the marital therapy procedures advocated in this book, it is included here as an additional source of support for these procedures.

BIRCHLER, G. R. Communication skills in married couples. In A. S. Bellack & M. Hersen (Eds.), *Research and practice in social skills training*. New York: Plenum, 1979.

Research is reviewed which supports the view that it is not specific problems but rather the communication skills and specific strategies employed for problem resolution that differentiate distressed from nondistressed relationships. The empirical literature specifically relevant to communication skills of married couples is thoroughly reviewed for both "enrichment" and "clinical" approaches. Communication skills are defined as the observable, trainable, verbal, and nonverbal behaviors concerning the way messages are sent and received between husbands and wives. It is concluded that although communication skills training (CST) is the most prevalent training procedure applied annually to thousands of couples seeking marital enrichment, few studies have incorporated comprehensive behavioral measures to validate this approach. However, taken together, the studies do indicate the efficacy of CST for the "enrichment" population. Similarly, the practice of CST in marital therapy is described and reviewed. Both the uncontrolled comparative group studies and the controlled outcome studies suggest fairly convincingly that systematic skill training approaches are generally superior to several more traditional forms of intervention for improving distressed couples' communication and marital satisfaction. The controlled outcome studies suggest further that the problem-solving component of CST in combination with contingency contracting is particularly effective in producing desirable behavioral and cognitive changes in distressed couples. At the end of the marriage enrichment and marital therapy sections is a discussion of the current status and future directions of these areas.

Index